ISBN: 978-0-9788603-7-0 Soft Cover
ISBN: 978-0-9788603-8-7 Hard Cover

Merritt, Hawkins & Associates Guide to Physician Recruiting

First Printing – April, 2007

Printed in the United States of America

Practice Support Resources, Inc., Publisher
Additional copies of this book may be ordered by calling 1-800-967-7790 or online at www.practicesupport.com.

About Merritt, Hawkins & Associates
Guide To Physician Recruiting

"This is a no-nonsense compact book brimming with information for recruiting doctors. It is based on 20 years of experience in the recruiting field and contains facts on the physician shortage, what doctors want, where they want to settle, what they expect in terms of salaries and benefits, and how to persuade doctors to join a group or hospital."

Forbes.com

"Every once in a while a book comes down the pike that is worth every cent you pay for it. Merritt, Hawkins & Associates Guide to Physician Recruiting is such a book. It contains information for recruiting doctors you won't find in such compact form anywhere else."

Richard Reece, M.D., Editor-in-Chief,
Physician Practice Options

"A detailed, strategic, and practical guide that is must reading for health care administrators, physician recruiters, practice administrators, and others interested in physician recruiting."

W. Vail Willis, Vice President,
Physician Services
LifePoint Hospitals, Inc.

Merritt, Hawkins & Associates
Guide To Physician Recruiting

By James Merritt, Joseph Hawkins, and Phillip Miller

Merritt, Hawkins & Associates
A Division of AMN Healthcare
5001 Statesman Drive
Irving, Texas 75063
800-876-0500
469-524-1400
www.merritthawkins.com

Acknowledgements

The authors would like to thank Mark Smith, Executive Vice President of Merritt, Hawkins & Associates, Kurt Mosley, Vice President of Business Development, and Lee Garber, Senior Vice President of Sales Operations, for their assistance and expertise in compiling information for this book. We also wish to thank Stephanie Godwin, Manager of Business Development, for the many hours she devoted formatting the book and creating the jacket design.

About the Authors

James Merritt

James Merritt co-founded Merritt, Hawkins & Associates, the nation's leading physician search and consulting firm, in 1987. Mr. Merritt also is co-founder of Staff Care, the nation's largest temporary (*locum tenens)* physician staffing firm, Med Travelers, a leading allied health care professional staffing firm, and RN Demand, a temporary nurse staffing firm. These companies, known as The MHA Group, merged with AMN Healthcare in 2005 to form the largest health care staffing company in the United States. An acknowledged health care staffing industry leader, Mr. Merritt has been cited in numerous publications, including *The Wall Street Journal, USA Today, Modern Healthcare, Hospitals & Health Networks* and many others. Mr. Merritt has written extensively on physician staffing issues and is co-author of the book *Will the Last Physician in America Please Turn Off the Lights? A Look at America's Looming Doctor Shortage.* Now in its third edition, the book has been referred to as a "must read" by Charles Lauer, publisher of *Modern Healthcare.* Originally from Toronto, Canada, Mr. Merritt now lives in Dallas, Texas.

Joseph Hawkins

Joseph Hawkins co-founded Merritt, Hawkins & Associates with Mr. Merritt in 1987 and also is the co-founder of Staff Care, Med Travelers and RN Demand. Throughout more than 25 years in the health care staffing industry, Mr. Hawkins pioneered many of the physician search and consulting methodologies commonly practiced in the field today. An acknowledged health care staffing expert, Mr. Hawkins has been cited in dozens of publications, including *Fortune, Inc., The Wall Street Journal, American Medical News, Modern Healthcare* and *Hospitals & Health Networks.* Mr. Hawkins has written numerous articles on physician staffing issues and is the co-author of the book *Will the Last Physician in America Please Turn Off the Lights? A Look at America's Looming Doctor Shortage.* Firms founded or managed by Mr. Hawkins have conducted over 30,000 physician search assignments throughout the United States. Raised in Miami, Florida, Mr. Hawkins now lives in Dallas, Texas.

Phillip Miller

Phillip Miller serves as Vice President of Corporate Communications for The MHA Group and AMN Healthcare. Mr. Miller has over 20 years of corporate communications and public relations experience and has been cited by *U.S. News & World Report, The Wall Street Journal, People Magazine, National Public Radio, USA Today,* and many other media outlets. Mr. Miller has authored or co-authored over 400 articles on health care staffing and other topics, and is co-author of the book *Will the Last Physician in America Please Turn Off the Lights? A Look at America's Looming Doctor Shortage.* Mr. Miller is from the Washington, D.C. area and now lives in Dallas, Texas.

Contents

CHAPTER 1

DOCTORS ARE DIFFERENT

The authors of this book are not physicians – and no, none of us has played one on television. But based on the thousands of doctors we have talked to, we feel safe in saying that physicians today are different, both from other professionals and from physicians the way they used to be 10 or 20 years ago.

Understanding these differences is a key to successful physician recruitment. You can not consistently identify appropriate physician candidates, create rapport with them, and convince them to relocate to your community unless you understand their unique concerns and challenges.

For this reason, not just anyone can be an effective physician recruiter, though some organizations operate as if this were the case. The U.S. Army, for example, simply reassigns nurse recruiters or recruiters of enlisted personnel to be physician recruiters, giving them a list of doctors to contact and a pat on the back. Even in the private sector, physician recruiters often have to fend for themselves without any formal training in their craft.

This stems in large part from the fact that physician recruiting is not an established profession requiring a degree or any national or local certification. Anyone with a rolodex and a phone can call themselves a physician recruiter. But without knowing doctors, they will not be consistently successful.

This book is dedicated to the proposition that physician recruitment is a distinct, challenging, and rapidly evolving profession requiring a wide knowledge base, a strong work ethic, and considerable powers of persuasion. There is an art to it, but there also is a science. It is not a realm for the unprepared or the unmotivated. How can it be when physician recruiters are expected to attract to their organizations or to their clients some of the most highly educated, motivated, and particular people in the world?

One Size Does Not Fit All

Consider that physicians are essentially scientists by temperament and training. They spend four years in college studying chemistry, biology and math, then four years in medical school, three or more years in residency training, and often an additional one to three years in a specialty fellowship. That's 11 to 15 years of college and post-graduate training.

Though all physicians have extensive training, they differ greatly in terms of what they do. There are now over 190 recognized medical specialties in which physicians can obtain board certification. Physicians in each specialty have varying concerns when it comes to evaluating practice opportunities: one size does not fit all. Nuances regarding the style of practice being offered, equipment available, nurse staffing, compensation and other issues often vary from specialty to specialty.

Listed below are some of the currently recognized medical specialties:

Recognized Medical Specialties

Abdominal Radiology
Abdominal Surgery
Addiction Medicine
Addiction Psychiatry
Adolescent Medicine
Adult Reconstructive Orthopedics
Aerospace Medicine
Allergy
Allergy & Immunology
Clinical Laboratory Immunology
Anatomic/Clinical Pathology
Anatomic Pathology
Anesthesiology
Blood Banking /Trans. Medicine
Clinical Cardiac Electrophysiology
Cardiovascular Diseases
Cardiothoracic Radiology
Chemical Pathology
Child & Adolescent Psychiatry
Child Neurology
Clinical Biochemical Genetics
Clinical Cytogenetics
Clinical Genetics
Clinical/Lab. Derm. Immunology
Clinical/Lab Immunology (IM)
Clinical/Lab Immunology (PED)
Clinical Molecular Genetics
Clinical Neurophysiology
Clinical Pathology
Clinical Pharmacology
Colon & Rectal Surgery
Cosmetic Surgery
Craniofacial Surgery
Critical Care Medicine (Anes)
Critical Care Medicine (IM)
Critical Care Medicine (OBGYN)
Cytopathology
Dermatology
Dermatopathology
Dermatologic Surgery
Developmental-Behavioral Ped.
Diabetes
Diagnostic Radiology
Emergency Medicine
Endo, Diabetes, & Metabolism
Endovascular Surgical Neuro
Gynecologic Oncology
Hand Surgery
Head & Neck Surgery
Hematology (Internal Medicine)
Hematology (Pathology)
Hematology /Oncology
Hepatology
Hospitalist
Immunology
Infectious Disease
Internal Medicine
Internal Medicine/Pediatrics
Interventional Cardiology
Legal Medicine
Maternal & Fetal Medicine
Medical Genetics
Medical Management
Medical Microbiology
Medical Oncology
Medical Toxicology (EM)
Medical Toxicology (Pediatrics)
Medical Toxicology (Prev. Med.)
Molecular Genetic
Molecular Genetic Pathology
Musculoskeletal Oncology
Musculoskeletal Radiology
Neonatal-Perinatal Medicine
Nephrology
Neurodevelop. Disabilities (PED)
Neurodevelop. Disabilities (Psy/Neuro)
Neurology
Neuroradiology
Neurological Surgery
Neuropathology
Neuropsychiatry
Neuroradiology
Nuclear Cardiology
Nuclear Medicine
Nuclear Radiology
Nutrition
Obstetrics
Obstetrics & Gynecology
Occupational Medicine
Ophthalmology
Oral & Maxillofacial Surgery
Osteopathic Manipulative Medicine
Pediatric Cardiothoracic Surgery
Pediatric Critical Care Medicine
Pediatric Dermatology
Pediatric Emergency Medicine
Pediatric Endocrinology
Pediatric Gastroenterology
Pediatric Hematology/Oncology
Pediatric Infectious Disease
Pediatric Nephrology
Pediatric Ophthalmology
Pediatric Orthopedics
Pediatric Otolaryngology
Pediatric Pathology
Pediatric Pulmonology
Pediatric Radiology
Pediatric Rehabilitation Medicine
Pediatric Rheumatology
Pediatric Surgery (Neurology)
Pediatric Surgery (Surgery)
Pediatric Urology
Pediatrics
Pharmaceutical Medicine
Physical Medicine & Rehab
Plastic Surgery
Plastic Surgery (Head & Neck)
Procedural Dermatology
Proctology
Psychiatry
Psychoanalysis
Psychosomatic Medicine
Public Health/General Preventive
Pulmonary Critical Care Medicine
Pulmonary Disease
Radiation Oncology
Radiological Physics
Radiology
Reproductive Endocrinology
Rheumatology
Selective Pathology
Sleep Medicine
Spinal Cord Injury Medicine
Sports Medicine (EM)
Sports Medicine (Family Practice)
Sports Medicine (IM)
Sports Medicine (Orthopedic Surgery)
Sports Medicine (Pediatrics)

Epidemiology
Facial Plastic Surgery
Family Medicine
Forensic Pathology
Forensic Psychiatry
Gastroenterology
General Practice
General Preventive Medicine
General Surgery
Geriatric Medicine (FP)
Geriatric Medicine (IM)
Geriatric Psychiatry
Gynecology
Orthopedic Surgery
Orthopedic Surgery of the Spine
Orthopedic Trauma
Foot & Ankle, Orthopedics
Otolaryngology
Otology/Neurotology
Pain Management
Pain Medicine (Psychiatry)
Pain Medicine
Palliative Medicine
Pediatric Allergy
Pediatric Anesthesiology (Pediatrics)
Pediatric Cardiology
Sports Medicine (Physical Med/Rehab)
Surgical Critical Care
Surgical Oncology
Thoracic Surgery
Trauma Surgery
Transplant Surgery
Undersea/Hyperbaric Med (EM)
Undersea/Hyperbaric Med (Preventive)
Urology
Vascular & Interventional Radiology
Vascular Medicine
Vascular Neurology
Vascular Surgery

The length, intensity and highly specific nature of their training distinguish physicians from most other professionals. In what other ways are physicians different?

No "Ladder To Success"

Generalizations are suspect, but in the course of close to 25 years in the physician recruiting field, there are certain broad statements we can make with confidence. One is that physicians do not approach their careers in the same way other professionals do. They typically are not seeking to climb the corporate ladder or "make partner." Contrary to popular perception, few doctors are attracted to medicine by the money. Intellectual curiosity and the unique power and appeal of the physician/patient relationship usually are the magnets that draw physicians to medicine.

As a result, physicians rarely move to advance their careers, as other professionals do. A title on the door or a pay raise are not particularly powerful inducements to most doctors. They are more likely to be attracted to a medical practice simply because it allows them to be doctors, or, these days, to be parents, hobbyists, and fully rounded individuals as well as doctors.

Reimbursement and Regulation

Physicians also are different from other professionals by virtue of the ground rules of contemporary medicine. These ground rules are largely determined by the way in which medical services are paid for in the United States today. Medicare sets physician payment rates for a wide range of services categorized as Diagnostic Related Groups (DRGs.) An orthopedic surgeon might be reimbursed $500 by Medicare for setting a simple bone fracture, and $1,000 for setting a compound bone fracture. Private insurance companies often set their reimbursement rates based on what Medicare pays.

The point is that physicians rarely set their own fees. Their fees are dictated to them by Medicare, Medicaid, HMOs, PPOs and other third party payers. The money reimbursed to them for services rendered may have little or no relation to their cost of doing business. What can be more aggravating is that sometimes third party payers also influence what physicians can or can't do for their patients, by declining to pay for services physicians may believe their patients need.

This is not the environment most of us work in. There is no "third party" barrier between the lawyer, the accountant, the computer programmer, the plumber, the mechanic and his or her clients. They all set a fee, perform a service, and are paid directly by the person for whom they did the work. Imagine a plumber who fixes a pipe for a fee set by the government – a fee that does not meet the cost of his tools. The plumber then submits a bill -- not to his client, but to an agency or insurance company. The agency or company then declines to pay the bill on the grounds that they do not cover that particular service under those particular circumstances.

It would be no surprise if, under these conditions, plumbers became a generally cranky group – especially if they had to complete 11 to 15 years of post-college training to become plumbers.

In addition, while most professionals must adhere to government or industry guidelines, they usually do not have nearly the level of regulation to deal with that doctors do. The federal tax code "only" runs to 11,000 pages, while the Medicare regulatory code by which doctors must abide is some 130,000 pages long. Doctors must document just about everything they do, or risk civil and criminal penalties for fraud and malpractice. When it comes to filling out documents and forms, just about every day for doctors is like tax time in early April is for the rest of us.

Moreover, when doctors make a mistake in the course of their duties (or when a patient *thinks* they made a mistake) they are quite likely to be sued. Unlike you and me, they can't make an error and then come in early to the office the next day to patch things up. Instead, their professional reputations may be put on the line and, even if the suit is completely without merit, they are in for some sleepless nights.

The Greatest Profession

Of course, doctors also are different from the rest of us for reasons that are positive. They can perform incredibly complicated, life enhancing surgery. They can deliver babies. They can (as one doctor recently did for one of the authors of this book) restore your sense of smell. They can stop death in its tracks, or they can ease a patient's passage from this world. Doing what they do, they have a unique perspective, from which they get to observe the human condition during the most dramatic and intense stages of life.

That's why there are so many more shows on television about doctors than there are about accountants, grocers, ad men or motivational speakers. That's also why even with all the hassles physicians complain about, medicine remains the greatest of professions.

In order to successfully recruit physicians, you must be able to walk in their shoes and see with their eyes. A Zen master would no doubt say, "You must ***be the physician.***"

We won't go that far, but it is important to realize that doctors are indeed different and that recruiting them is an art and a science unto itself. In the following pages we will discuss both the subjective aspects of recruiting physicians – the art – and those specific, measurable activities that lead to success – the science.

It begins with an understanding of something we call "the iceberg effect." This is the proposition that much of the effort and expertise that goes into a successful physician search takes place "beneath the surface," an idea we explore further in Chapter Two.

CHAPTER 2

THE ICEBERG EFFECT

Like a finished product on a shelf or in a showroom, there is more to a successfully completed physician search than meets the eye. A shiny new car on a lot, for example, began with a carefully arrived at design. Raw materials had to be gathered from a variety of sources, tools configured to shape the materials, a team of experts assembled to put the parts together, and transportation arranged to bring the vehicle to the market. The product itself is merely the tip of the iceberg relative to the time, effort, resources and expertise that went into making it.

From a recruiting standpoint, a newly recruited physician represents the tip of the iceberg. He or she is the shiny car patients see on the "showroom" floor. What patients don't realize (or necessarily care about) is the time, effort, resources and expertise that went into putting the physician in place.

That is not their concern. But it is very much the concern of anyone tasked with the job of recruiting doctors. Recruiters must understand the necessary, sequential steps that lay the groundwork for success. The diagram below illustrates the iceberg analogy. Another way to convey the concept is through the old military maxim: "the battle is won or lost before the first shot is fired."

The Physician Recruiting "Iceberg"

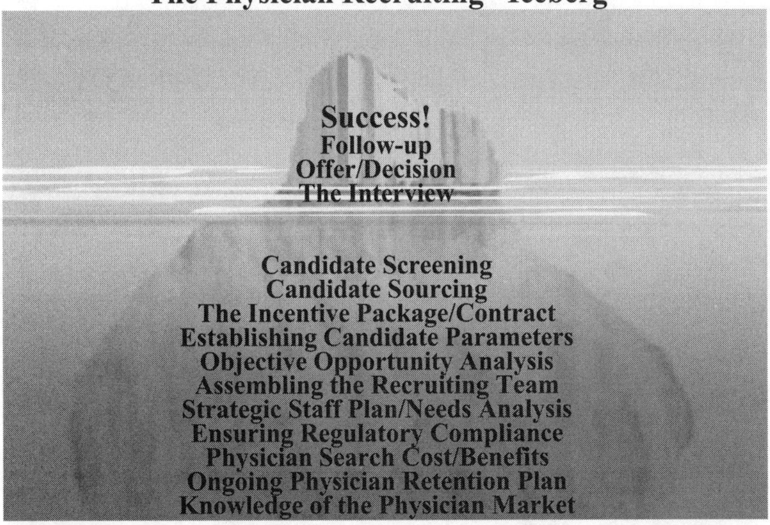

The principal reason why many physician search efforts fail is that a preponderance of emphasis is placed on the elements at the tip of the iceberg and not enough attention is paid to the elements that comprise the iceberg's foundation. Recruiters often hear hospital or medical group administrators say, "Just find me candidates, we'll know what to do from there."

But physician search is a sequential process and it is difficult to succeed when steps in the process are omitted or ignored. "Just getting a physician" is not as simple as it sounds. For one thing, you have to know what you are getting into, the same way you would if you went on an expedition for a valuable commodity of any kind. What is the market like for what you seek? Will it be hard to find? Who else is looking? What are the legalities involved? What is our game plan? Who is on our team? What are the costs and benefits? What resources do we need to accomplish the task at hand?

All of these questions should be answered before recruiters have their first conversation with potential candidates. A good place to begin is with a brief look at the current market for physicians, a subject we examine in Chapter Three.

CHAPTER 3

THE PHYSICIAN MARKET

Someone who is smarter than we are once said: "Without doctors, hospitals are just empty hotels with bad food."

Even with all the changes that have taken place in medicine in recent years, doctors remain at the center of health care delivery. The most powerful tool in health care is not a gamma knife or an MRI; it is the physician's pen. Without a doctor's signature, patients do not get admitted or discharged from a hospital, prescriptions cannot be written or filled, and equipment won't be ordered or used.

Indeed, physicians drive the lion's share of the $2 trillion health care economy. And, despite the proliferation and the importance of a wide range of allied health care professionals, physicians still perform the diagnosis and procedures that are at the core of health care delivery.

It is hardly surprising that their services are in demand. But how great is the demand for doctors, and how large or small is the corresponding supply? It's a simple question, but the answer is of paramount importance to anyone involved in physician recruiting.

The Physician Shortage

There are still a few academics and health care analysts who argue that the U.S. has a sufficient number of physicians. For the most part, however, academics, health analysts, organized medicine and the media have finally realized that America is in the midst of a serious, wide-spread, and protracted physician shortage.

This is not a point we will address in much detail in this book – not because it isn't important, but because we addressed this issue in a previous book entitled *"Will the Last Physician In America Please Turn Off the Lights? A Look at America's Looming Doctor Shortage."*

In that book we outlined the reasons for the physician shortage and how it is affecting health care delivery. We won't repeat our arguments here in any depth or include much data supporting them. But it is important to stress that ***every phase of physician recruitment*** – from retention, to cost considerations, to the candidate you ultimately select – must be based on the fundamental understanding that the U.S. has too few doctors.

The table below offers one widely noted projection of physician supply and demand in the U.S. through the year 2020. According to this projection by Richard "Buz" Cooper, a noted professor at the University of Pennsylvania, the U.S. will be short 200,000 physicians within about 15 years.

Physician Supply/Projected Shortages Through 2020

	1929	2000	2010	2020
Total Physicians	144,000	772,000	887,300	964,700
Physicians per 100, 000 pop.	119	270	283	280
Pop. in millions	121	286	325	335
Shortage of physicians	N/A	N/A	50,000	200,000

Source: Cooper, et al, Health Affairs, Feb. 2002

The majority of academics and analysts who track physician supply – many of whom met at a conference in May, 2005 in Washington, D.C. sponsored by the Association of American Medical Colleges (AAMC) – concur that the physician shortage is going to build in the coming years and will not be resolved anytime soon. Edward Salzberg, Director of the AAMC's Center for Workforce Studies, who addressed the conference, noted that even if the number of U.S. medical school graduates could be increased by 15% immediately, the shortage of physicians by 2020 could exceed 200,000. In a subsequent meeting held in 2006, the AAMC resolved to increase U.S. medical school enrollment by 30%

Dr. J. Edward Hill, former president of the American Medical Association, wrote in the February 20, 2006 issue of *American Medical News* that the looming physician shortage "is no less ominous" than the threat of a pandemic.

Why has the physician shortage become such a major concern? Though we wrote a book addressing this question, the answer is quite simple. The supply of physicians in the United State is shrinking at the precise moment when demand for medical services is surging. The problem was once localized to mostly rural areas, but no longer.

Merritt, Hawkins & Associates, which was founded in 1987, used to work mostly in small to medium sized towns – places that traditionally have had a hard time recruiting physicians. Today, over 40% of the search assignments we represent are in communities of 100,000 or more. In the past, there were certain areas, mostly coastal towns and popular resorts, which never felt the need to engage a physician search firm such as ours. Today, it is not unusual for our company to represent medical groups and hospitals seeking doctors in some of the most popular resort destinations in the country – including the Florida Keys, Palm Springs, Aspen, the Napa Valley and Hawaii.

In addition, the "name brands" of the health care industry – renowned medical institutions which are immediately recognizable even to non-health care professionals – rarely if ever required the services of physician search firms in the past. Medical directors at these institutions had plenty of physician CVs on their desks to choose from. Today, even the name brands are finding it challenging to recruit the physicians they need and are using the services of physician search firms to assist them.

The competition for physicians in most specialties is intense and the overall supply situation is worrisome. For this reason, Merritt, Hawkins & Associates' parent company, AMN Healthcare, the nation's largest health care staffing firm, is underwriting research and advocacy conducted by a newly formed group called ***The Council on Physician and Nurse Supply.***

This group of well known and respected health care leaders is co-chaired by Richard "Buz" Cooper, M.D. and Linda Aiken, RN, Ph.D., both of whom are academics at the University of Pennsylvania. Members include leaders from the American Hospital Association, the Medical Group Management Association, Duke University, Emory University and other prestigious institutions. Its goal is to suggest ways in which the supply of physicians and nurses can be adjusted, and to help create the political will necessary to implement its recommendations. AMN Healthcare has committed considerable resources to funding the Council because the shortage of physicians and nurses has become so acute it is detrimental to the health care staffing industry, its clients, and the communities they serve.

A Sense of Urgency

At the risk of beating a dead horse, we'll repeat one more time that physicians are a precious commodity. There are not enough of them to go around. Physician recruiting incentives, candidate parameters, and, most importantly, the ***sense of urgency*** with which a search is conducted must begin with this premise.

Understanding the current imbalance between the demand for physicians and available supply is Physician Recruiting Market Knowledge 101. Market knowledge also embraces a number of other factors such as the federal rules governing physician recruitment, current levels of physician compensation, physician demographics and related topics, each of which is addressed separately in subsequent chapters.

Before addressing these topics, however, it is necessary to pose this question: Knowing how difficult doctors are to recruit today, what are hospitals and medical group administrators doing to ***retain the physicians they already have?*** A vital building block to any physician recruitment effort, one that also is at the base of the recruiting iceberg, is a strategic physician retention program that both secures current doctors and makes a hospital or medical group more attractive to prospective new physician candidates.

Prior to discussing how to bring new physicians to an organization, we will discuss methods for holding on to the ones you have.

CHAPTER 4

PHYSICIAN RETENTION

Physicians are the lifeblood of any hospital, medical group or other health care organization. Retaining them should be a top strategic priority for organizations committed to maintaining quality services and financial stability. Nevertheless, other priorities – reimbursement, community relations, emergency preparedness – often can crowd out the importance hospital and medical group executives place on the ongoing, daily task of maintaining positive physician relations.

When this is the case, physician recruitment becomes a matter of ***reaction*** rather than ***pro-action,*** as hospitals or groups must respond to the physician defections or abrupt retirements that take place within unstable staffs. Poor retention leads to gaps in service, which can have a negative effect on patient satisfaction. It also leads to losses in revenue that can amount to thousands of dollars per physician, per day. To this opportunity loss must be added the expense of physician recruitment (see Chapter 5) which can be wasted when doctors who have been recently recruited decide to leave.

Physician retention has become more problematic in recent years as medicine has shifted from the small, private practice model to the mid-to-large group practice model and the hospital employment model. Rather than being independent, small business owners, many physicians now are employed by medical groups or hospitals.

Younger physicians in particular are attracted by settings where they can be employees and do not have to deal with the billing and other administrative hassles of private practice, as well as the financial risks. It is generally easier for employed doctors to "pull up stakes" and move on than it is for those in private practice, who have employees counting on them and who have the deeper financial and psychological ties inherent to practice ownership. Consequently, the physician workforce has become more mobile.

This trend was quantified in an article published in the May 22, 2001 issue of *The New York Times,* which indicated that before 1990, only one to two percent of physicians changed jobs throughout a 20-year career. Ten years later, more than 10 percent of physicians changed jobs in any given year.

A study conducted by the Department of Health Science at Towson University in the 1990s examined turnover rates among younger, primary care physicians. The study looked at employed primary care physicians younger than 45 who had been in practice between two and nine years. The study showed that over a five year period, 55% of these physicians had left the practice in which they were originally employed. Twenty-percent of physicians in the study group had left two employers in five years.

Penn State Geisinger Health System in Danville, Pennsylvania also looked at physician retention issues in the 1990s while developing a physician retention plan for its multispecialty group practice of some 1,000 physicians.

Penn State Geisinger estimated that ***physician turnover rates range from 10% to 15% nationally.*** Larger medical groups and hospitals with which Merritt, Hawkins & Associates works generally report physician turnover rates ranging from six to ten percent. Penn State Geisinger's research showed that a variety of factors lead to physician turnover. The most significant factors include:

Causes For Physician Turnover:

*Lack of physician "fit" with partners and the practice environment
*Lack of clear communication of expectations to physicians ***during recruitment***
*Absence of two-way communication between physicians and practice management
*Failure to include physicians in the decision making process
*Lack of appreciation/recognition of physicians.

In our experience another leading cause of turnover, particularly in smaller medical groups, has to do with compensation. Usually, this is tied into factor two above – incoming physicians' expectations regarding how much they will earn and how income will be distributed in the group conflict with the reality of earnings and dollar distribution.

Communication is the Key

The importance of retaining physicians clearly increases as the number of available physician candidates decreases and as Generation X and Y physicians become more inclined to move from one practice to another.

Physician retention begins with good communication, a virtue that is often commended but just as often ignored.

For example, several years ago, our firm recruited a neurosurgeon to a community in the Upper Midwest who appeared to be a good fit for the medical group and the hospital. In touching base with him some months after placement, however, the physician indicated that he planned to leave the area. After he had practiced in the community for six months he was asked to attend a dinner that included another neurosurgery candidate who was being recruited to the group. Although the first neurosurgeon was very busy and would have been happy for the call coverage and potentially supportive of the recruitment, he was upset because nobody had discussed this recruitment with him. He mistook the lack of communication to mean that the group was unhappy with him and had decided to recruit a replacement. Instead of waiting for a termination letter from the group, he decided to be proactive and found another opportunity offering similar financial potential and a reasonable call schedule with a group that he felt he could trust to communicate with him regarding issues of importance, such as recruiting.

This anecdote illustrates a common cause of physician defection. While a great deal of effort, time and money typically are put into getting a physician to a community, there is a tendency to neglect physicians after arrival. This neglect often can extend to established members of the medical staff who seldom get the attention lavished on new candidates who are being wooed.

A cardinal rule of retention that recruiters know well is that ***physicians are not pulled from their practices as often as they are pushed.*** Recruiters generally are not able to lure doctors away from one practice to another with a range of tempting incentives such as big salaries or immediate partnership in a practice. Rather, we find physicians who are discontented with their current practice and are attracted by the promise of better conditions elsewhere.

The case for good physician communications is well stated by Thomas Kramer, president and CEO of Deaconess Health System, who was quoted in a study conducted by The Governance Institute as follows:

"When you need the goodwill of physicians, it is too late to create it. My advice: get ahead of competition by having a really good relationship with your doctors."

**Source: The New Competitive Landscape, 2003, The Governance Institute*

A Medical Staff Survey

An effective physician communication process includes both formal and informal components. A key formal component is a medical staff survey that should be conducted at least once a year. The survey can have a number of uses. First, it can provide a way to "take the temperature" of the medical staff. How satisfied are physicians with their practices and what can the hospital do to help?

A medical staff survey also can be a key element in an overall medical staff plan designed to determine how many additional physicians a community needs (see Chapter 7 for a discussion on medical staff planning). A sample medical staff survey is included below. This is a general boilerplate that should be amended as appropriate.

Medical Staff Survey
Sample Survey Instrument

Introduction:

General Hospital (or General Medical Group) is committed to meeting the needs of our medical staff. We would like to learn more about the challenges you face, the staffing, equipment, and operational needs you would like to see addressed, and how we may be able to assist you with these and other matters.

Please take a moment to complete the enclosed survey and return it in the postage paid envelope that has been provided. You may take the survey anonymously, or include your name and contact information if you would like results of the survey sent to you. Please complete the survey and return it by (insert date.) We greatly appreciate your consideration and look forward to assisting you.

Your name (optional): ______________________
Your specialty (optional): ______________________
Would you like results of the survey sent to you? Yes___ No___
If yes, please include your contact information:
Address______________________
Email______________________

1. What type of practice are you currently in?

☐ Solo ☐ Two Physician Group ☐ Three physicians or more ☐ Hospital based

2. What type of medicine do you practice?

☐ Primary Care ☐ Surgical Specialty ☐ Diagnostic Specialty ☐ Other

3. Which of the following best describes your current practice?

☐ I am too busy ☐ I am not busy enough ☐ I am as busy as I want to be

4. Which best describes your current feelings about your practice?

☐ I am very satisfied with my practice
☐ I am somewhat satisfied with my practice
☐ I am somewhat dissatisfied with my practice
☐ I am very dissatisfied with my practice

If you have an office based practice, about how many patients do you see in your office a month? __________ *(enter patient count)*

5. Is this an appropriate number?

☐ Too few
☐ Too many

6. How far are you booked out for (non-emergent) new patient appointments?

☐ Same Day ☐ 1 week or less ☐ 2-3 weeks ☐ 4-6 weeks
☐ 7-8 weeks ☐ 9-10 weeks ☐ 11-12 weeks ☐ 13 weeks or more

7. Do you have trouble referring your patients to local physicians?

☐ No, local physicians usually can see my patients in a timely manner
☐ Yes, it is often difficult for my patients to schedule timely appointments with local physicians

8. How long does it take to schedule your patients when you refer them to the following types of physicians?

	1 week or less	2 weeks	3 weeks	4 weeks	5 weeks	6 weeks
Family Practice	□	□	□	□	□	□
Internal Medicine	□	□	□	□	□	□
Pediatrics	□	□	□	□	□	□
General Surgery	□	□	□	□	□	□
Orthopedic Surgery	□	□	□	□	□	□
Cardiology	□	□	□	□	□	□
Gastroenterology	□	□	□	□	□	□
Dermatology	□	□	□	□	□	□
Urology	□	□	□	□	□	□
Add others as appropriate	□	□	□	□	□	□

9. Please consider medical services in our area. How would you rate the need for additional physicians in the following specialties?

	No Need	Need in 1-2 years	No need for 2+ years
Family Practice	□	□	□
General Internal Medicine	□	□	□
Pediatrics	□	□	□
General Surgery	□	□	□
Orthopedic Surgery	□	□	□
Radiology	□	□	□
OB/GYN	□	□	□
Gastroenterology	□	□	□
Cardiology	□	□	□
Add others as appropriate	□	□	□

10. How would you rate the need for additional physicians in your own practice?

□ No need now
□ I would like to add an associate within the next 12 months
□ I would like to add an associate within the next 12-24 months
□ Other ______________________________

11. When do you plan to retire?

□ Within the next six months
□ Within one year
□ 1-2 years
□ 3-4 years
□ 5 years or more

12. Rate the hospital in the following areas:

	Excellent	Good	Average	Poor
Patient registration	□	□	□	□
Patient discharge	□	□	□	□
Medical records	□	□	□	□
Operating rooms	□	□	□	□
Pathology/lab	□	□	□	□
Emergency room	□	□	□	□
Diagnostic Imaging	□	□	□	□

13. In what ways can the hospital assist you?

□ Marketing the Practice
□ Physician recruitment
□ Managed care contracts
□ IT support
□ Other ______________________

Thank you for your participation. Should you have any questions about this survey or wish to discuss it, please contact (*name of medical director or physician liaison.*)

The medical staff survey should be sent to physicians with a cover letter signed by the chief medical officer or other physician leader who enjoys the respect of the staff. The letter should encourage physicians to complete the survey and suggest that it presents an opportunity for them to influence hospital policy and have their voices heard.

In addition to the survey, hospitals can establish other formal physician communication channels. One is a physician advisory council composed of five to 10 unofficial physician leaders who meet with the hospital CEO once every two months or on some other suitable time frame. The council can serve as a sounding board for the CEO and as a conduit for physician opinions and concerns. A hospital staff newsletter, which can be sent out by email, is another formal communications method.

Informal communications methods also are important. Some hospitals hold regular "pizza and talk" sessions during which physicians are invited to share their ideas and concerns with administrators over lunch.

A key element (though, again, an often under-utilized one) is an open door policy. Administrators must make accessibility an ingrained behavior. Be where doctors are – join them in the lunch room, the operating room and visit the ER. Avoid the bunker mentality that leads to distrust and disillusionment among the medical staff.

Employ the Physician

Physician staffing trends tend to run in cycles. During the high tide of managed care, hospitals scrambled to acquire physician practices and to employ as many primary care gatekeepers as they could. Ultimately, the employment model didn't work for most hospitals and many lost money trying to manage employed physicians.

Now, physician employment is making a comeback, but with a twist. Often, it is physicians who are approaching hospitals seeking employed positions. Just as often, it is surgical and diagnostic specialists, not primary care physicians, who are making these requests. Fed up with high malpractice rates, the grind of running a practice, and the financial risks involved, specialists are seeking the relative simplicity and security of employment.

Ironically, it is hospitals that now have to be persuaded to take on physician employees (in some states, hospitals are barred from directly employing physicians). Burned during the physician practice management craze, hospitals are reluctant to go through the same process again. While this is understandable, we have repeatedly observed that employment is an increasingly attractive option for many physicians. In our experience, those hospitals that offer employed settings often enjoy an advantage over those that do not.

In order not to lose physicians to attractive, employed positions, more hospitals are at least exploring the idea of employing physicians themselves. We believe that employment will become an increasingly important recruitment and retention tool in coming years and will help address the problem of direct physician/hospital competition.

Pay Specialists for ED Coverage

In some communities, lack of medical specialist coverage in the ER is becoming an issue of critical importance. According to a 2006 national survey conducted by The Schumacher Group, a Lafayette, Louisiana-based emergency medicine management firm, 34% of hospital emergency department managers indicate that lack of specialty coverage in the ER poses a serious threat to patient safety.

The unfortunate fact is that physicians are increasingly unwilling to shoulder the malpractice risk and lifestyle burden of covering the ER without compensation. According to the Schumacher survey, 31% of hospitals now are paying physicians to cover the ER. Facilities that offer such compensation enjoy an enhanced recruiting posture and may also enjoy retention benefits.

Below is a breakdown of hourly rates for on-call pay per several medical specialties:

Specialty	In-House	Off-Site
Anesthesiology	$80	$32
Emergency Medicine	$72	-
OB/GYN	$85	-
Primary Care	$45	-
Psychiatry	$75	$18
Surgery	$48	-
Surgical Specialties	$81	$31
Trauma	$95	-

Source: Sullivan, Cotter and Associates On-Call Pay Survey

Gain Sharing/Joint Ventures

Aligning physicians financially with the hospital has proven to be a sound retention policy for some facilities. Gain sharing, which is the process of rewarding physicians for savings they achieve for the hospital, is an intriguing idea, and one which appears to be gaining the acceptance of government regulators.

In 2005, Pinnacle Health System's Harrisburg, Pennsylvania facility was cleared to standardize the use of 16 hospital supply items, and then share the cost savings with cardiologists. Given continued government approval, gain sharing will grow in importance as a physician retention tool.

The case for joint venturing with physicians is succinctly stated by the phrase: "A percentage of something is better than a percentage of nothing." If physicians are going to build a competing free-standing clinic or specialty hospital, it often is better to "join 'em if you can't lick 'em." According to the October 22, 2002 edition of *Healthcare Financial Management,* more than half of the freestanding heart hospitals in the country involve some level of participation or sponsorship by a not-for-profit organization.

With "skin in the game," physicians are more likely to ensure the efficient use of resources and to insist on staff productivity. It remains to be seen, however, the extent to which federal and state regulations may limit physician ownership of and referrals to joint ventures.

The Primacy of the Workplace

Next to good communications, the most important physician retention tool is a quality work environment. Hospitals evaluating their physician relations and retention plans should keep in mind the "primacy of the workplace." The work environment – its accessibility, efficiency, the benefits it offers patients – is paramount to most physicians.

Susan Whitley, M.D., put it this way in an article in the April 15, 2002 issue of *American Medical News:*

"It's not that referring physicians prefer ambulatory surgery centers. But we prefer a quick treatment and an effective treatment in a safe environment."

Joseph Wasserman, President and CEO of Lakeland Regional Health System, echoed this sentiment in The Governance Institute study referenced earlier:

"A few doctors may be motivated by avarice and greed, but most are looking to compete because they are unhappy with the current levels of service in the hospital for both patients and doctors."

There are a variety of ways to enhance the hospital work place from the physician's perspective – though few of them are particularly easy or cheap.

They include:

- Ensuring a qualified, appropriate nursing staff. A key irritant to many physicians is lack of appropriately trained nurses
- Improving physician access to patient data
- Enhancing test turnaround times
- Ensuring timely, consistent OR availability
- Timely, efficient patient admissions/release
- Convenient parking/access for physicians
- Enhanced ER triage/patient turnaround
- Implementing a hospitalist program

Though these measures are not quick fixes, most of them align with patient needs and requests, and will better position hospitals for the emerging era of consumer driven care. In addition, physicians stand to benefit more from efficiency gains at an existing facility than they do from their return on investment in a specialty hospital, as the graph below indicates:

ROI vs. EFFICIENCY GAINS

♦ Average doctor investment in a specialty hospital:	$10,000 - $50,000
♦ Annual return:	30%
♦ Annual take-home:	$3,000 - $15,000
♦ Efficiency gains leading to one more ORs case per week:	$6,000/mo.
♦ Annual increase in physician income:	$72,000

Source: The New Competitive Landscape, The Governance Institute, 2003

The key is to create an efficient, patient-oriented environment that, to the greatest extent possible, allows physicians to do what they are trained to do. This will enhance their peace of mind, and, in many cases, grow the size of their pocketbooks, as well.

It will also make life harder for physician recruitment firms or competitors to take doctors away. When a hospital is well run and both physician and patient oriented, it is a lot more difficult for recruiters to persuade physicians that the grass is really greener on the other side.

Once you have looked inward and implemented a proactive and ongoing physician retention program to keep the doctors you have, it is time to focus outward again and consider bringing in new physicians. An important question to ask – one that should be asked at the base of the "recruiting iceberg" – is how much is this effort going to cost relative to the potential benefits it will bring?

We take a closer look at this question in Chapter Five.

CHAPTER 5

UNDERSTANDING COSTS/BENEFITS

Though physician recruiting has a profound impact on a wide range of hospital operations, the cost of this activity often is not fully understood or accurately quantified. How much money does it take to attract and retain a doctor, how can these costs be minimized, and what is the expected return on investment?

By obtaining answers to these questions, one can gain insight into the physician recruiting process and help ensure that hospitals and medical groups are following the most effective and cost efficient recruiting methods.

The costs of physician recruiting will vary by medical specialty. Supply and demand trends differ among specialties and obviously some types of physicians command higher salaries than others. In general, however, recruiting costs break down as follows.

- *Physician salary/income guarantee.* A hospital or medical group's largest financial exposure in physician recruiting usually is represented by the salary or income guarantee offered to attract physician candidates. Whether the physician is directly employed by the hospital, is employed by a group practice, or is established as a solo physician in the community, the hospital usually will front the salary or guarantee needed to attract the physician to the service area. The chart below shows the average annual base salary or income guarantee offers made to physicians in eight different medical specialties, as tracked in Merritt, Hawkins & Associates 2007 Review of Physician Recruiting Incentives. ***Note: A Copy of the 2007 Review is included at the end of this book.***

Average Base Salaries/Guarantees Offered to Physicians

Cardiology	$391,000
Orthopedic Surgery	$413,000
Internal Medicine	$174,000
OB/GYN	$247,000
Family Practice	$161,000
Gastroenterology	$365,000
General Surgery	$301,000
Urology	$400,000

Source: 2007 Review of Physician Recruiting Incentives, Merritt, Hawkins & Associates

These numbers reflect the base financial package offered to recruit physicians, and do not include signing bonuses, benefits, production bonuses, CME, educational loan forgiveness or other perks. Given these additional incentives, the investment needed to attract physicians either out of training or from an established practice can be considerable.

- *Staff or recruiter time and fees.* Many hospitals employ full-time, in-house physician recruiters. Others use full-service retained physician search firms and/or contingent "headhunters" to attract physicians, sometimes as a supplement to in-house recruiting staff. Salaries and fees associated with recruiter time can vary greatly. In-house physician recruiters often earn a base of $35,000 to $65,000 and may receive bonuses based on number of placements made. Recruiter fees can range from $15,000 to over $30,000 per placement.

- *Candidate sourcing.* Certain medical specialists – cardiologists, orthopedic surgeons, gastroenterologists – are in unprecedented demand today. Thousands of hospitals and medical groups are vying for a limited number of physicians, increasing the difficulty and cost of finding candidates. Today, a number of sourcing methods – journal advertising, networking, direct mail, the Internet – must be employed continuously to identify suitable physician candidates. The expense of this activity can range from $5,000 to over $15,000 per search.

- *Interviewing.* Hospitals and medical groups generally pay all the costs associated with a physician interview. Travel, accommodation and entertainment costs usually range from $1,500 to $3,000 per interview.

- *Relocation.* This is another variable cost depending on where the physician is relocating from. The average relocation allowance in the 3,000 plus physician searches Merritt, Hawkins & Associates conducted from March 31 of 2006 to April 1 of 2007 was $9,808.

- *Practice marketing.* Hospitals and medical groups often pay to announce the opening of a new physician's practice and help introduce the physician to the community. Practice marketing costs can range from a few hundred dollars to several thousand.

Combined, these factors can drive the potential cost of one physician search to $400,000 or more, as illustrated in the table that follows.

Potential Cost of a Cardiologist Search

Physician income guarantee/salary	$390,000
Benefits/perks	$50,000
Recruiters fees (in-house or agency)	$25,000
Candidate sourcing	$10,000
Candidate/spouse interview	$3,000
Physician Relocation	$10,000
Practice Marketing	$3,000
Total	$491,000

"Hidden Costs"

In reviewing these costs it is apparent that while the expense of identifying, interviewing, and relocating candidates can be considerable, the hospital's greatest financial exposure is associated with physician salaries/income guarantees and benefits. Should a newly recruited physician prove unsuccessful in his or her practice and be unable to sustain a patient base or a meaningful level of referrals, the hospital or group may be unable to recoup the physician's salary or income guarantee. Most frequently, lack of physician success occurs because there was not a sufficient need for the physician in the hospital's service area. However, in some cases when the need in a particular specialty is questionable it may still make sense for a hospital or group to move forward with recruitment. Breaking even or taking a loss on an individual practice in order to pay a competitive salary may make sense if the physician can generate enough referrals, ancillary studies, admissions, etc. to generate overall positive revenue for a hospital or group.

The first key to minimizing financial exposure in physician recruiting, therefore, is to accurately assess the need for a given medical service in the community ***prior to*** recruiting a physician to provide that service. (See Chapter 7 for a discussion of the various methods by which hospitals can determine the need for physicians in their service areas.)

Once a need for a physician has been established and a search initiated, it is important for the search to be conducted efficiently. Poor search methodologies lead to wasted motion, principally through the interviewing of inappropriate candidates, which needlessly prolongs the process and increases costs.

It also should be considered that there is a significant "hidden cost" of recruitment that takes place when a position on the medical staff goes unfilled. Each day in which a physician is not in place seeing patients can lead to both a loss of patient loyalty and to a loss of revenue.

The graph below illustrates the average net inpatient and outpatient revenue physicians in various specialties generate for their affiliated hospitals.

Average Annual Income Generated by Physicians For Their Affiliated Hospitals

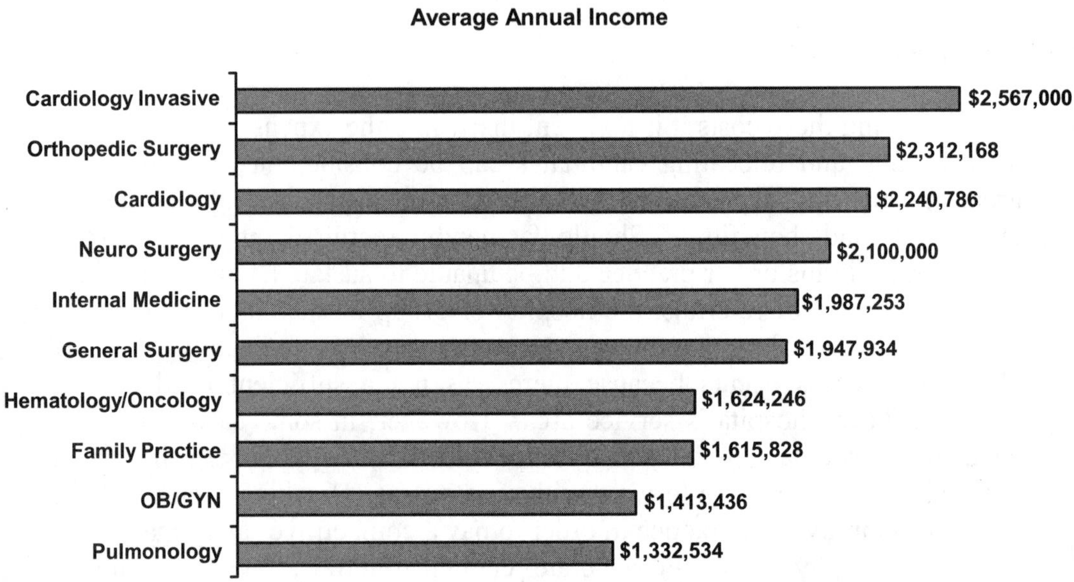

Source: Merritt, Hawkins & Associates' 2007 Physician Inpatient/Outpatient Revenue Survey

These numbers were derived from a survey Merritt, Hawkins & Associates conducts of hospital chief financial officers nationwide. **A copy of this survey is included in this book.** On average, physicians generate $1.5 million a year in inpatient and outpatient revenue for their affiliated hospitals. Each month that a needed physician is not in place can cost a hospital $100,000 or more. The cost to recruit a physician, therefore, is minimal relative to the potential financial benefit, even if the physician only stays for a limited amount of time.

Of course, from a patient care perspective, there is no dollar value that can be placed on the physician's skills and expertise. It is the physician's clinical ability and knowledge that allows a hospital or medical group to fulfill its mission to the community and this benefit obviously is well understood by hospital and group administrators and by the medical staff.

Wasted motion and hidden costs can be avoided by ensuring that a search is structured in such as way that communication, contractual matters, candidate sourcing, screening and interviewing are all mapped out on the front end. Methods for structuring a search for success (and cost effectiveness) are reviewed in subsequent chapters of this book.

First, however, it is necessary to consider another way in which physician recruiting can be very costly. If the physician recruitment process is conducted in a manner that is not compliant with federal regulations, the penalties may include both steep fines and even jail time for those involved.

Before a physician search is initiated, and before we proceed to other topics, the issue of compliance must be addressed.

CHAPTER 6

COMPLYING WITH PHYSICIAN RECRUITING REGULATIONS

Until the mid-to-late 1980's, physician recruitment in the United States was a largely unregulated activity. That is not the case today, however. The Internal Revenue Service, the Department of Health and Human Services, and the "Stark Law" all have imposed requirements governing how physician recruitment must be conducted and the conditions under which recruiting incentives may be offered.

We are not attorneys, but as physician recruiters we do have to keep a close eye on federal physician recruiting regulations, and we work with legal professionals who are experts in this area. In this chapter we do not offer legal advice, but we do outline some of the legal issues pertaining to physician recruitment that attorneys at national law firms specializing in health law have conveyed to us. Keep in mind that all physician recruiting contracts should be reviewed by an attorney well versed in this area of the law and that the following does not constitute legal advice.

Recruitment and The IRS

The Internal Revenue Service has a stake in physician recruitment when it is being conducted by tax-exempt hospitals. The IRS is concerned that private individuals do not benefit financially from their relationship with not-for-profit entities, which potentially could happen in physician recruitment. Should such illegal "inurement" take place, a hospital could stand to lose its not-for-profit status.

Through a series of memorandums beginning in 1986, the IRS established that a hospital's tax exempt status would not be adversely affected if the physician recruiting agreement is structured properly. The agreement must be structured in such a way that any benefits accruing to the new physician are *incidental to* the benefits the new physician is providing to the hospital's community. One way to demonstrate that the new physician is providing significant benefits is to show that he or she will be meeting a demonstrable need in the community for additional medical services of the type which the recruited physician provides.

On April 21, 1997, the IRS released Revenue Ruling 97-21. This ruling postulates five physician recruiting scenarios and outlines what incentives can be offered in each case. Generally speaking, the greater the need in the community, the more that can be offered to recruit a physician. Based on circumstances, Ruling 97-21 establishes that hospitals may offer the following to physician recruits:

- ♦ An income guarantee
- ♦ A signing bonus
- ♦ Malpractice insurance for a limited period
- ♦ Office space for a limited number of years at below market rent
- ♦ A mortgage guarantee on the physician's home
- ♦ Financial practice start-up assistance
- ♦ Reimbursement of moving expenses
- ♦ Malpractice "tail" coverage

Again, there must be a need for the physician in the community, all incentives offered must be "reasonable" based on current market standards, the recruitment agreement must be in writing, and the recruiting agreement should have the blessing of the hospital's Board of Directors. It also should be noted that the ruling focuses on non-employee physicians. Should the hospital hire the physician as an employee then it simply must ensure that no more than "reasonable compensation" is paid to the physician.

Revenue Ruling 97-21 is very useful in that it established for the first time direct legal precedent that physician recruitment by tax-exempt hospitals is a perfectly appropriate charitable activity. It also illustrates that the IRS will consider physician recruiting by tax-exempt hospitals on a case by case basis in which "continuum of need" is a deciding factor. The greater the need for the physician, the more latitude a hospital has in offering incentives.

The "50 Percent" Rule

Prior to issuing Revenue Ruling 97-21, the IRS entered into a closing agreement with Hermann Hospital in Houston, Texas. The 1994 agreement included a clause prohibiting Hermann Hospital from paying more than 50 percent of the recruiting costs on behalf of an existing medical group. Though the Hermann ruling was not intended to set a legal precedent, many hospitals felt limited by this part of the Hermann agreement and reduced the assistance they were providing in cases where they were helping an established group in the community to recruit a physician.

Revenue Ruling 97-21 supersedes the Hermann Agreement, however, and does not contain the so-called "50 percent" rule. In addition, we are aware that at least one hospital has received a private letter ruling from the IRS in which it is specifically stipulated that hospitals are not limited to funding only 50 percent of the recruitment to an existing group.

This subject also is relevant to the discussion of the Stark recruiting regulations and is pursued further below.

The Federal Illegal Remuneration Statutes

The federal government, pursuant to Section 1128B(b) of the Social Security Act, prohibits the payment of "remuneration" to any person in exchange for the referral of government program patients to health care facilities for services that may be paid by the government programs. Hospitals, for example, are prohibited from paying physicians for referrals of Medicare or Medicaid patients. The payment of recruiting incentives to physicians potentially could be construed as an inducement to refer such patients to the recruiting hospital. Hospitals engaging in this practice risk criminal and civil fines, criminal prosecution, and the loss of their right to participate in Medicare and Medicaid programs.

Since the statute is rather broad, the administrating agency (the Department of Health and Human Services) was directed by Congress to identify practices that will not be subject to prosecution or provide the basis for Medicare/Medicaid exclusion. A final Safe Harbor regulation for physician recruitment was effective as of November 19, 1999.

The Safe Harbor applies to for-profit and not-for-profit hospitals and is limited to hospitals recruiting physicians (i) to Health Professional Shortage Areas (HPSAs), which includes many rural areas and certain underserved urban areas, and (ii) who have been practicing within their specialty for less than one year. The payment of recruiting incentives to physicians who are relocating to a HPSA or who have been practicing for less than one year will be afforded Safe Harbor protection as long as the following seven standards are met:

Seven Safe Harbor Standards

- The arrangement is set forth in writing
- The new physician, if already in practice, must not relocate from less than

100 miles from the location of the new practice, and at least 85% of revenue in the new practice must be generated by new patients

- Benefits provided to the physician shall not exceed three years and can't be substantially renegotiated during that time
- The physician shall not be required to refer patients to the recruiting hospital
- The physician shall not be restricted from establishing privileges at other hospitals
- Benefits to physicians cannot be based on the volume of referrals they make
- The new physician will agree to see Medicare and Medicaid patients

Since this Safe Harbor applies primarily only to HPSA hospitals, there is still some gray area regarding acceptable physician recruiting practices for hospitals in non-HPSA areas, which would include most urban area hospitals, under the federal illegal remuneration statute. Until such time as the rules are clarified, all hospitals are advised to consider the seven Safe Harbor standards in structuring physician recruiting arrangements.

The Stark Law

The "Stark Law," named after its sponsor, Congressman Fortney "Pete" Stark, states that physicians cannot refer Medicare and Medicaid patients to hospitals in which they have a financial interest, which can be either through ownership or compensation. Payments made by a hospital to recruit a physician are considered compensation subject to the Stark Law. Regulations promulgated under the Stark Law, which were effective July 26, 2004, create an exception to the basic prohibition in the case of physician recruitment if:

- The recruitment arrangement and its terms are in writing and signed by both parties
- The physician is not required to refer patients to the hospital
- The amount of financial assistance is not tied to the volume or value of any patient referrals the physician may make to the hospital
- The physician is not barred from establishing privileges at another hospital or from referring to another hospital

Final regulations implementing Phase II of Stark were released by the Center for Medicare and Medicaid Services (CMS) in September, 2007. The new regulations include provisions applicable when a hospital is recruiting a physician to join an existing group. Among other requirements, the regulations include the following:

Medical groups recruiting physicians with the assistance of a hospital may in some cases impose a non-compete agreement on the incoming physician. Non-competes may be permissible in states where such agreements are part of state law. This represents a change over initial regulations promulgated in 2004, which prohibited medical groups from imposing a non-compete on new physician recruits if the group was receiving financial recruiting assistance from a hospital.

In addition, if the hospital pays recruiting fees to an outside recruiting firm directly to carry out the search, and does not pay any amount to the group or the incoming physician, the group may require the newly recruited physician to sign a non-compete. Other physician recruiting regulations established by Stark include:

- A hospital funding recruitment to an existing group can only pay for "additional incremental expenses" that accrue to the group because of the new physician. It cannot pay for a pro-rated share of the group's fixed overhead expenses, such as office rent, equipment, or personnel, unless such expenses are a direct result of the new physician joining the group. It should be noted, however, that the new Stark regulations released in 2007 create an exception to this rule. In a case where a group in a Health Professional Shortage Area or rural area is replacing a deceased, retiring, or relocating doctor, the hospital ***can*** pay for a pro-rated share of the group's fixed overhead expenses, such as office rent, equipment or personnel, not to exceed 20% of the practice's aggregate costs.

- Groups must maintain and provide evidence of incremental expenses resulting from the presence of the new physician for five years.

- Incoming physicians must relocate to the geographic area served by the hospital, which is defined as all of the contiguous zip codes from which the hospital's inpatients are drawn when the hospital draws fewer than 75% of its patients from contiguous zip codes.

- The physician must relocate their practice (not their home) 25 miles, or derive at least 75% of revenues in the new practice from new patients. An exception is made for physicians coming out of residency or for those who have participated in their specialties for less than one year. Exceptions also may be made for physicians completing military obligations and for others who don't have an established patient base.

A Step Forward

The new Stark regulations of 2007 can in general be viewed as an improvement over the 2004 version of Stark from a physician recruiting perspective. In those states where non-compete clauses are permissible, groups may be able to protect themselves against potential future competition from newly hired physicians. This should make groups more open to collaborating with hospitals on physician recruiting. In our experience, many groups became reluctant to recruit when they could not longer impose a non-compete on physicians joining the group while receiving financial recruiting assistance from a hospital. This forced some hospitals to recruit into solo practice settings, which is difficult to do in today's environment, and undermined to some extent the symbiotic relationship between medical groups and hospitals that can be important to physician recruiting success.

The 2004 Stark regulation limiting hospitals to providing only "additional incremental expenses" presented a serious challenge for many hospitals. The rule is intended to eliminate any financial benefit that physicians already established in a community may gain when a hospital assists them to recruit physicians. In discussions our firm has had with Center for Medicare and Medicaid Services (CMS) officials, it is clear this rule was implemented to prevent physician recruiting abuses such as those alleged to have been committed by a for-profit facility in San Diego. The hospital was criminally charged with violating the federal anti-kickback law for offering physician relocation agreement monies to local groups in exchange for patient referrals.

A problem arises, however, when an existing group loses a physician. In the past, a hospital could assist an established medical practice to find a new physician by providing a salary or guaranteed income to the incoming physician and allocating to the new physician a pro rata share of existing office space, equipment, personnel, and other expenses associated with the new physician's practice for one year.

That arrangement was prohibited by Stark in 2004, so that an established group or a physician that lost a partner due to death, retirement or relocation would see overhead increase by as much as 50% and could get no relief from the hospital. The hospital was virtually obliged in such instances to recruit a new physician into a ***solo practice setting***, in which case it could assist the new doctor with expenses such as office space rental, personnel and equipment. Since very few physicians are willing to work solo, particularly in smaller or rural communities, the 2004 rule made recruitment that much more difficult and did not reflect the realities of physician recruitment today.

However, CMS agreed with the objections to this rule that Merritt, Hawkins & Associates submitted to it and modified the rule as referenced above for groups located in Health Professional Shortage Areas or rural areas. This restores a key recruiting arrangement for medical groups and hospitals in mostly rural areas (and some urban areas) and is encouraging proof that government agencies do listen and respond to concerns from those in the field.

Dealing with Stark II

In light of the new rules, we suggest the following:

♦ Eliminate all non-competes from physician employment agreements when the hospital is assisting an established group to recruit if such agreements are not permissible in the state. If they are permissible, structure them in accordance with state law and with the guidance of qualified legal advisors.

♦ Should a physician practicing in an existing group in the hospital's service area relocate, retire or pass away, the group should consider immediately reducing clinical and administrative staff if it is not located in a medically underserved area. Such staff may be rehired in the event that a new physician is added, requiring the presence of more staff, which would be an additional incremental expense for the recruited physician. If the group is located in a medically underserved area or a rural area, these steps will not be necessary.

♦ When a newly recruited physician arrives, he or she should obtain their own health, malpractice, and disability insurance, hire their own staff, purchase their own equipment, and contract with outsourcing services for billing and related functions. This demonstrates that additional expenses are directly attributable to the presence of the new physician. Again, an exception occurs for groups in medically underserved areas that have lost a physician to death, retirement or relocation.

- ♦ Recruit residents, physicians who have been in practice less than one year, or physicians from outside the hospital's service area. Since residents and new physicians do not have an established patient base, they cannot be induced to refer patients to the hospital, unlike established physicians in the community who do have a patient base. The new Stark regulations released in 2007 expand the list of physicians who do not have an established patient base to include military physicians completing their obligations and others.

- ♦ Follow all the federal rules pertaining to physician recruitment. These include demonstrating a need in the community for a new physician, paying a salary or income guarantee that is "reasonable," ensuring the agreement is in writing and is approved by the hospital Board, allowing the physician to obtain privileges at other hospitals, requiring that the physician see Medicare patients, and offering incentives without any requirement that the physician refer patients to the hospital.

The Stark regulations released in September of 2007 include a number of provisions not directly discussed in this book and should, like all regulations pertaining to physician recruiting, be reviewed by attorneys experienced in this area of the law.

What You Should Not Do

In light of IRS, HHS Safe Harbor, and Stark Regulations, the following is a list of things hospitals should not do when recruiting physicians.

- ♦ Tie compensation to referrals in any way
- ♦ Recruit from across town (except medical residents and others without an established patient base)
- ♦ Pay established physicians a stipend to recruit new doctors
- ♦ Pay for non-incremental expenses when assisting an established medical group to recruit (unless the group is in a HPSA or a rural area and has lost a physician to death, retirement, or relocation)
- ♦ Limit physicians from establishing privileges at other hospitals
- ♦ Pay physicians beyond what is "reasonable"

What You Can or Should Do

- ♦ Craft a policy statement/resolution of the Board of Directors on physician recruitment

- Put in writing your awareness of the rules and your commitment to follow them
- Make recruitment contingent on community need
- Conduct a formal physician community needs analysis plan
- Put the physician recruiting agreement in writing
- Specify the services the physician will provide
- Specify benefits that will be provided to the physician
- Pay physicians what is "reasonable" by current market standards
- Get Board approval for physician agreements
- Consider employing the physician (assuming permissible under any state corporate practice of medicine restrictions)
- Require physicians to treat Medicare/Medicaid patients
- Recruit residents or physicians outside of the community
- Let physicians establish privileges where they wish
- Have your physician recruiting policies reviewed by competent attorneys

Though there are still grey areas, the basic rules of physician recruitment are fairly simple and well established. The government acknowledges that physician recruitment is a necessary activity but remains nonetheless sensitive to hospitals overpaying recruited physicians (or the groups they join) or paying them for referrals.

Knowing what your needs are and being able to demonstrate them is an important part of the equation and is the subject of the next chapter.

CHAPTER 7

DEMONSTRATING COMMUNITY NEED FOR PHYSICIANS

How can a hospital demonstrate that it has a need for additional doctors?

As mentioned in Chapter 6, answering this question is central to any effort to comply with IRS, HHS and Stark related physician recruiting regulations. However, a community needs assessment plan has other benefits. A thorough plan with a sound methodology:

- ♦ Provides a pro-active, strategic blue-print to follow
- ♦ Creates buy-in for recruitment among the current medical staff
- ♦ Assesses the demographics and practice patterns of current staff
- ♦ Shows potential recruits that there is a documented need for their services

Without a medical staff plan, hospitals and medical groups are obliged to rely on the ***"Little Dutch Boy"*** approach to physician recruitment. A physician will retire or abruptly leave the community, creating a "hole in the dam" which the hospital or group will try to fill. This largely reactive posture creates stress and a lack of continuity of services. It is preferable to know what kind of physicians you are going to need in the short to mid-term and then plan and allocate resources accordingly.

In addition, recruitment is a major political bone of contention between hospitals and the medical staff. Existing physicians can torpedo a search if they feel there is no need for a new doctor or if they believe their opinion was not asked. By soliciting physician input through a medical staff plan, recruitment can become, in effect, the staff's idea.

A staff plan provides a guide to who your medical staff is, their style of practice, retirement plans, etc. It also can be used to demonstrate to incoming physicians that there is a need for their services in the community. A plan which indicates that 90% of local physicians support the recruitment of a new doctor and that the service area has grown by 30% makes a strong statement about the need for a doctor in the community. A hospital or group that can point to such a plan will have more credibility with candidates than a hospital or group lacking such data.

In the past, hospitals and groups often had few objective yardsticks to measure community need for physicians. They would simply tell us, "We just know we need a cardiologist." Today, many facilities have an objective methodology for demonstrating a need for additional physicians. What constitutes such a methodology?

The IRS offered an indication in Physician Recruitment Guidelines released in October, 1994 as an attachment to the closing agreement entered into with Hermann Hospital referenced in Chapter 6. The Guidelines indicate that a physician will not be a "permissible recruit" unless there is a demonstrable community need for the physician, as evidenced by:

1. A physician to population ratio as suggested by the Graduate Medical Education National Advisory Committee (GMENAC) that is deficient in the specialty being recruited

2. Demand for a particular medical service in the community coupled with a documented lack of availability of the service or long waiting periods for the service, if the physician is being recruited to increase availability of that service

3. Federal designation of the community at the time of the recruitment agreement as a Health Professional Shortage Area (HPSA)

4. A reasonably expected reduction in the number of physicians of that specialty serving the hospital's service area due to the anticipated retirement within the next three year period of physicians presently in the community

5. A documented lack of physicians serving indigent or Medicaid patients within the hospital's service area, provided that newly recruited physicians commit to serving a substantial number of Medicaid and charity care patients

The Hermann Hospital Agreement has since been superseded by Revenue Ruling 21-97 released April 21, 1997, but the methods for determining community need as listed in the Guidelines remain valid, if incomplete.

Elements of A Community Needs Assessment Plan

In order to confirm community need for physicians, the elements above and other factors should be included in a formal Community Needs Assessment Plan or Medical Staff Plan. Such a document verifies the need for additional physician services, and serves as part of a hospital's efforts to comply with federal physician recruiting regulations. It can be used in case of a government audit to demonstrate the rationale for physician recruiting. It also can be used as an effective recruiting tool because it objectively demonstrates to physician recruits that a need for their services exists.

Physician-to-Population Ratios.

Physician-to-population ratios are one of a variety of elements in a comprehensive physician needs assessment plan. The most well known of these ratios are the GMENAC ratios alluded to above. Some ratios, such as GMENAC's, are "needs-based" and reflect the projected need for medical services in the population based on the researchers' theoretical models of per capita health care consumption. Others are "visits-based," such as the ratios compiled by Hicks & Glenn, researchers at the University of Missouri.

Visit-based ratios look at federal government statistics indicating how many annual visits to a particular type of physician a population of 100,000 typically generates. They then divide into this the number of annual patient visits that a physician in that specialty typically sees, as tracked by the Medical Group Management Association. For example, if 100,000 people typically generate 75,000 visits to a family physician each year, and each family physician sees 2,500 patients annually, then the "right" number of family physicians is 30 per 100,000 people.

Physicians Required Per 100,000 Population

Following are suggested estimates for the number of physicians required per 100,000 population, as indicated by three different sources.

SPECIALTIES:	GMENAC	GOODMAN	HICKS & GLENN
Primary Care			
Family Practice	25.2	N/A	16.2
Internal Medicine	28.8	N/A	11.3
Pediatrics	12.8	N/A	7.6
Medical Specialties			
Allergy/Immunology	0.8	1.3	N/A
Cardiology	3.2	3.6	2.6
Dermatology	2.9	1.4	2.1
Endocrinology	0.8	N/A	N/A
Gastroenterology	2.7	1.3	N/A
Hem/Onc.	3.7	1.2	N/A
Infectious Disease	0.9	N/A	N/A
Nephrology	1.1	N/A	N/A
Neurology	2.3	2.1	1.4
Psychiatry	15.9	7.2	3.9
Pulmonology	1.5	1.4	N/A
Rheumatology	0.7	0.4	N/A
Other Medical Specialties	N/A	N/A	N/A
Surgical Specialties			
General surgery	9.7	9.7	4.1
Neurosurgery	1.1	0.7	N/A
OB/GYN	9.9	8.4	8.0
Ophthalmology	4.8	3.5	3.2
Orthopedic surgery	6.2	5.9	4.2
Plastic surgery	1.1	1.1	2.3
Urology	3.2	2.6	1.9
Other Surgical Specialties	N/A	N/A	N/A
Hospital Based			
Emergency Medicine	8.5	2.7	N/A
Anesthesiology	8.3	7.0	N/A
Radiology	8.9	8.0	N/A
Pathology	5.6	4.1	N/A
Pediatric Subspecialties			
Pediatric Cardiology	N/A	N/A	N/A
Pediatric Neurology	N/A	N/A	N/A
Pediatric Psychiatry	N/A	N/A	N/A
Other Pediatric Subspecialties	N/A	N/A	N/A

Clearly, the ratios vary widely in their recommendations. Three separate ratios put the need for psychiatrists per 100,000 population variously at 15.9, 7.2, and 3.9.

Each of these ratios has its adherents and detractors. GMENAC met only once and promulgated its ratios over 25 years ago. Though its numbers are over two decades old, they are still commonly referenced in medical staff plans. The fact that GMENAC ratios pre-date the proliferation of managed care and that the population has aged considerably since 1980 only partly explains why these and other ratios are problematic. The real reason they are not definitive is that they suggest standardization is achievable in the patchwork of health care markets in the United States that make up a vast heterogeneous whole.

Consider. Can the same ratio of cardiologists-per-population really apply in young, largely immigrant South Texas and in old, largely geriatric sections of South Florida? Clearly, these disparate populations are as unlikely to utilize medical services at the same rate as they are to purchase pizza, hair coloring, or shoe polish at the same rate.

Physician-to-population ratios, then, are only a signpost or general indicator of physician need, rather than a definitive benchmark. A reliable projection of community need for physicians requires a thorough analysis of local conditions, including:

Physician Counts

Exactly how many physicians are practicing in the service area already – not just on the recruiting hospital's staff, but in total? ***No projection of current and future physician need can be accurate without this core data.*** Deriving an accurate physician count can be difficult, however. Some physicians may split time in two different service areas, and so cannot be considered full-time-equivalents (FTEs) in either area. Family physicians or internal medicine practitioners may be providing OB or cardiology services, and therefore are neither FTEs in primary care nor in the specialty they are crossing into. Residents may also contribute services without being considered FTEs.

The only way to conduct an accurate physician count in some medical markets is to profile each physician's practice, usually through telephone canvassing of the physicians or their office administrators. Only by doing so can you obtain a more or less definitive view of how many true FTEs are in the area. Short of this, a scrupulous attempt must be made to count physicians by examining the hospital's staff roster, the local phone books, and AMA listings of physicians in the area. Keep in mind that just because a local physician is not on the recruiting hospital's staff does not mean he or she is not providing services to the community. What is being measured in a community needs assessment plan is the needs of the community, not necessarily of the hospital.

Physician Demographics

How old are established physicians and when are they likely to retire? How many residents are on the staff? How many female physicians? The latter is an important consideration as female physicians on average work 18% fewer hours a week than male physicians, according to the AMA. In addition, anecdotal evidence suggests that female physicians retire at an earlier age than male physicians. A comprehensive community needs assessment plan will include a breakdown of local physician demographics.

Physician Input

Local physicians usually have the best insight into local demand for medical services. Physicians know if there are long wait times to schedule their patients with specialists. They also know which specialty services their patients need that currently are not available in the community. A survey of established physicians (such as the sample provided in Chapter 4) can reveal how busy they are relative to national averages, whether their practices are open to certain populations such as Medicare patients, and what recruitment needs they see in the community.

In our experience, physicians often are conservative in their assessment of how many new physicians are needed in their communities. If more than 50% of physicians surveyed indicate that a particular specialist is needed then it often can be inferred that a need exists. A physician survey also allows physicians to participate in the medical staffing process, building a consensus that can be essential during physician recruiting. Physicians usually are less likely to resist physician recruiting initiatives when their opinion has been asked and considered.

Patient Demographics

Is the local population growing? What segments are growing the fastest? Medicare patients utilize some medical services at three times the rate of younger populations, so patient aging is a key factor. Which are the geographic areas of fastest growth? What level of insurance and access to health care services does the population have? Is language a barrier to care? These and other questions pertaining to patient demographics must be answered to accurately gauge physician need.

Disease Incidence

Health care challenges differ from region to region. Cardiovascular disease is rampant in some areas of the Midwest, while skin cancer rates often are high in sunny, coastal areas. Hospital admissions data and other statistics can reveal how local disease incidence varies from national averages and may provide a rationale for recruiting physicians who can address local health care needs.

HPSA Designations

A federal designation as a Health Professional Shortage Area (HPSA) offers a strong indication that there is a need for additional physicians in a community. However, HPSA designations only indicate a shortage of primary care physicians and psychiatrists. A HPSA designation will not necessarily support the need for a surgical or diagnostic specialist, which must be supported by additional data.

Portrait of Need

From this combined data, a portrait will emerge of the local service area, showing the number, age and practice patterns of established physicians, current patient demographic trends, disease incidence and areas of immediate and long-term physician need. Physician-to-population ratios can add depth or perspective to this picture.

The final document should be updated annually to ensure accurate physician counts and related information. While useful in the event of an audit of physician recruiting practices, a comprehensive physician needs assessment plan also can be a working tool offering strategic direction and marketing data for hospital administration. The plan should conclude with a specialty-by-specialty analysis that sums up the general data and indicates what recruiting steps should be taken, if any. The chart below provides a hypothetical example.

Specialty By Specialty Analysis of Need

Internal Medicine

FTE Count	♦ 2.75 in MSA
Ratios	♦ two show a deficit, one a surplus
Physician Demographics..	♦ two IMs 55 or older, one female IM
Physician Practices	♦ all IMs see more patients than MGMA average
	♦ all scheduled three weeks out
	♦ one planning to retire
	♦ one wants to add an associate
Physician Survey	♦ 75% of existing staff sees an immediate need for IM
Patient Demographics	♦ largely geriatric population
Disease Incidence	♦ high incidence of diabetes
HPSA	♦ No
Action Item	♦ begin immediate search for two IMs, two more in next 24-36 months

With a data driven staff plan in place, a hospital or medical group is in position to initiate those search requirements identified as being the most immediately pressing.

Who is responsible for formulating and executing the physician search plan? Physician search is not a solo endeavor. It requires a group of people with a common goal working together – the Recruiting Team.

CHAPTER 8

RECRUITING TEAM, ASSEMBLE!

As we have discussed, a variety of factors have come together to make physician recruiting a relatively more complex, challenging and strategic activity than it has been in the past.

For compliance reasons alone, many hospitals are establishing medical staff development (MSD) committees to ensure that physician recruitment is conducted in a manner consistent with federal guidelines and to promote board participation and approval. Such committees also serve a variety of other purposes, however. Tasks delegated to MSD committees typically include:

- Working with current staff on succession planning
- Working with current staff on retention and satisfaction issues
- Establishing recruitment goals and recommendations
- Involvement in the Medical Staff Development Plan, including selection of a consulting firm, participation in the planning process, approval of the final plan and presentation of the plan to physicians, the board and the community at large.
- Working with the hospital CEO to establish physician candidate education, experience and related parameters
- Providing input regarding recruitment incentives, financial packages and contracts that will ultimately be approved by the hospital's board
- Active involvement in the recruitment process and selection of outside recruiting firms, if necessary
- Reviewing candidate CVs during the recruitment process
- Participating in candidate interviews
- Approving the offer that is needed to obtain candidate commitment
- Participating in any post-relocation social events and meetings to welcome and introduce new physicians to the community

In order to be effective, MSD committees need to be comprised of appropriate members dedicated to achieving clearly understood goals. The first task is to determine who will be on the committee.

Committee Make-Up/Reporting

MSD committees vary in size, membership and reporting structure from hospital to hospital, based on the size of the facility and what the committee is charged with doing. MSD committees usually range from 4 to 10 members. In virtually all cases, the Chief Medical Officer is a member of the committee. In addition, the acting Chief of Staff is either a member or attends meetings to represent physicians at large. The Medical Staff Coordinator also usually is a member of the committee but is not always granted a vote.

The central figure and leader of the committee, however, is the hospital CEO or medical group administrator. In physician recruiting today, active CEO participation is critical to both setting goals, establishing candidate parameters, ensuring responsiveness, and driving negotiations to a successful close.

Members of the MSD committee variously include:

- Board members (with an emphasis on physicians)
- Staff physicians, usually a representative sample of specialties and medical groups
- Chief Executive Officer or Group Administrator
- Physician recruiter
- Chief Medical Officer
- Chief Nursing Officer
- Chief Financial Officer
- Hospital department representatives from Community Relations, Marketing, Strategic Planning, and Patient Care

Care should be taken to appoint committee members who have a long-term interest in the viability of health care in the community rather than those who have a short-term interest or a particular vested interest (i.e., a physician who is anxious to recruit a partner, or, conversely, a physician anxious to forestall recruiting efforts.)

If the committee is given the final authority to determine recruitment priorities, rather than just making recommendations to the Board, some legal advisors suggest that physicians on the committee abstain from voting on recruitment decisions that would affect their own specialty or group.

Another way to avoid potential conflicts of interest is to structure the committee so that physicians do not have the majority vote.

Reporting structures, like committee membership, may vary from case to case. In some instances, the MSD committee is a sub-committee of the Board, in others it is part of the medical staff structure. In some hospitals, the MSD committee serves as an advisory group reporting directly to the CEO.

Setting the Agenda

Though MSD committees may vary somewhat in terms of their purpose, make-up and reporting structure, they all need a specific agenda to follow in order to achieve targeted goals. Generally, the committee's purpose is to lay the strategic foundation for both overall physician relations and physician recruitment.

As previously discussed, an initial priority in today's market is to retain the physicians you have. The MSD committee can be essential to this effort by acting as a bridge to current staff physicians so that the hospital understands their future plans and their current needs and concerns. In particular, the committee can approach staff physicians regarding retirement or relocation, so that a strategic succession plan can be put in place. The committee also can help staff physicians work through issues such as call coverage, potential physician-hospital competition, allied staffing, equipment requests or other matters that can lead to physician dissatisfaction.

The MSD committee has a further mission when it comes to selecting physician leaders. The committee can help identify candidates for medical directorships or other executive positions within the hospital, paving the way for more physician involvement in administration – a crucial step in addressing the rising level of physician-hospital conflict prevalent in health care today. The MSD committee therefore has an important role to play whether or not the hospital is actively recruiting physicians.

When recruitment is initiated, the committee is responsible for helping to demonstrate that a need for additional physician services exists. Again, this usually requires that a thorough physician needs assessment be conducted, either by hospital personnel or by an outside firm. Whoever conducts the assessment, the MSD committee must be satisfied that the methodology used provides a truly objective analysis of the service area that will be credible in the eyes of the medical staff, physician recruitment candidates, and potential federal auditors. The committee then usually helps determine what kinds of physicians should be recruited and how they should be recruited. Some members of the committee may participate directly in the recruitment process.

The need for physician recruitment is not always manifest to all stakeholders, and the need to offer recruitment incentives is sometimes even less apparent, particularly to members of the Board who are not health care professionals. The committee chairman, who should be a hospital representative, may wish to educate committee members about the current physician supply and demand situation by sharing articles or books regarding the physician shortage, or even inviting consultants educated on the market to address the group in person. This will underline the fact that physician recruitment is very challenging today and that a concerted recruitment effort is necessary to attract most types of physicians. Any committee member with decision making power must be educated on the current state of the physician market so that decisions are not reached in a vacuum.

The MSD committee also needs to be satisfied that incentives being offered to physician recruits are "reasonable" by market standards, as IRS, HHS and Stark laws require. The committee should be provided with physician compensation data similar to the data presented in Chapter 11 of this book so that it has an understanding of what incentives are both reasonable and competitive today.

The MSD committee should help determine what types of physician candidates will be considered. When setting candidate parameters, it is important to focus on the essentials. Ivy League trained physicians with movie star charisma are in short supply. Good training, a positive bedside manner, good communications skills, a strong work ethic and a true desire to relocate to the hospital's service area should trump more superficial issues such as personal appearance, "star quality" or country of origin. This important topic is addressed in more detail in Chapter 10.

The objective is to generate broad-based consensus from diversified stakeholders without suffering "death by committee." In order to avoid inertia, the committee must be able to vote with a quorum.

The Search Process

The MSD committee establishes a broad consensus for the need to recruit physicians and ensures that incentives are reasonable and transparent with no payment for patient referrals stated or implied. All this is in accordance with federal recruiting regulations. Committee members are often directly involved in candidate interviews, hospital/clinic tours and other details that are of particular interest to candidates and their spouses, such as local schools and hobbies.

Continual communication with physician candidates is crucial. Faulty communication before or after the candidate interview is a principal reason why many search efforts fail (this subject is addressed in more detail in Chapter 16.). If members of the MSD committee are readily available as needed to answer questions, then communication can be an asset. However, it is best to limit the number of people contacting candidates before and after interviews to one or two to ensure that a consistent message is conveyed.

As physician search becomes more challenging and more closely scrutinized by government agencies, it is evolving into a larger, more collaborative effort involving hospital administration, the medical staff and the community. An effective medical staff development committee helps tie these elements together into a focused and compliant whole.

CHAPTER 9

AN OBJECTIVE PRACTICE/COMMUNITY ANALYSIS

Those who are susceptible to Cupid's arrows know how easy it is to fall in love. For some, love and marriage come easy, and for others Cupid is not so quick to strike.

But the question in marriage -- and in physician recruitment -- is not just who ***you*** will fall in love with but ***who will fall in love with you?***

In both cases, an objective self-examination is in order. If you are planning to propose to someone with movie star looks and Bill Gates' money, you will have to bring quite a bit to the table yourself. It's good to have self-esteem, but in seeking a prospective mate you have to be realistic about what you offer if you hope to enter into an enduring match.

Similarly, in forming a physician recruitment plan, hospitals and medical groups must take an honest inventory of what the practice and community have to offer in the context of what else is available in the great buyer's market that most physicians benefit from today. Civic pride is certainly a virtue, but it should be considered that people everywhere take pride in their communities, including people in communities who may be vying for the same physicians that you are. Consider that physician candidates already may have visited five communities very similar to yours.

To the greatest extent possible, you must walk through the practice and community in the physician's shoes, seeing it through the eyes of potential candidates. That is why Merritt, Hawkins & Associates insists on conducting an in-depth, on-site opportunity analysis of the physician search assignments that we represent, so that our recruiters can view each opportunity the way a physician will see it.

We also are very cautious about assigning recruiters to searches located in communities where they grew up. While they have the advantage of knowing their "home towns," it also is possible that they will be too emotionally tied to their community to be objective. The principle is born out in other professions such as law, where attorneys hire lawyers to represent them in their own legal affairs, and in medicine, where physicians will see other doctors when they need their own illnesses diagnosed.

Examining the Practice

The medical staff plan documents why a need exists for a new physician, but it does not document the features and benefits of each opportunity. If you are shopping for any high ticket item, such as an automobile, you want to know everything about it – miles per gallon, warranty, safety features, etc. before you make a purchase. A good salesperson will give you all the facts about the car – the strengths and weaknesses – before demonstrating the vehicle in an actual test run.

In the same way, whoever is representing a practice opportunity should know all the features and benefits that are likely to be of interest to physician candidates. This information should be gleaned during the opportunity analysis.

In reporting to the MSD committee, the recruiter should know the following:

♦ *Why are you recruiting?* Again, a rationale for the recruitment should be included in the medical staff plan. It is up to the recruiter representing the opportunity to be familiar with the plan. Anecdotal reasons such as "our community is growing," or "the doctors say they are really busy," are generally insufficient for data-driven physicians who, after all, often are being asked to leave one practice for another, while uprooting their families in the process.

There is an old saying in science: "Extraordinary claims require extraordinary proof." The extraordinary claim you are making is that your practice opportunity is better than the one a physician candidate is in now, or is better than the other opportunities he or she may be considering. It is much more effective to say that family physicians in your community are handling 40% more ambulatory patient encounters than the MGMA average than to say "our physicians are really busy."

♦ *How long has a need for a particular physician existed?* The first question people ask in buying a house is, "how long has it been on the market?" If it has been on the market a long time, why? Physician candidates examining your opportunity will ask the same question. If an opportunity has been open six months or more, it may raise red flags. Is there a lack of support for the search among local physicians or other political problems? Is the financial offer below market rates in the specialty? An objective opportunity analysis should reveal answers to these questions so that changes to the recruiting strategy can be made, if necessary. It is important to have honest answers to share with physician candidates, such as: "Dr. Smith initially did not support the search, but he has since revised his views. You will be meeting with Dr. Smith personally on the interview and I am confident he will express his enthusiasm about having you on the medical staff." Again, it is easier to adjust on the front end of a search rather than waiting until the "tip of the iceberg" stage referenced in Chapter 2.

♦ *Patient volume.* Recruiters should know the prospective patient volume of the practice opportunity, both inpatient and outpatient. How many patients are established physicians in the community seeing? How many patients are leaving the community for services the new physician will be providing?

In addition to asking about patient volume, physician candidates will ask the simple question: "Who are my patients going to be?" Community demographic information regarding population growth, age, gender, and economic factors will be necessary to answer this question, as will data about patients of the practice the new physician may be joining.

♦ *Payer mix/reimbursement rates.* While the "golden age" of fee-for-service medicine may be over, some places have more "gold" in them than others. From a payer perspective, the United States is a patch quilt, not a uniform blanket. Payer mix varies considerably from region to region and a positive payer mix can be a major incentive that will attract physicians from other regions or states. High levels of employment leading to high levels of private insurance, relatively high Medicare reimbursement rates, minimal capitation/managed care, and low Medicaid volumes all can persuade physicians that the grass really is greener on the other side. A positive payer mix with relatively high reimbursement rates should be quantified and emphasized. Recruiters in an area with a less positive payer mix should be able to explain why, a mediocre payer mix notwithstanding, high patient volumes, low overhead or other factors enable physicians to make a competitive income in the area. Of course, income is just one issue. A favorable payer mix also means more practice autonomy and a better chance that physicians will be able to treat patients as they see fit.

♦ *Collection rate.* Physicians are looking for efficiency in a practice and a minimum of administrative hassles. As mentioned earlier, that is one reason why many doctors are seeking employed settings. A high collection rate signals an efficient practice where the constant grind over getting paid has been minimized or eliminated. Recruiters should be able to document collection rates in existing physician practices and describe the back-office functions that allow practices to enjoy favorable collections. These could include electronic medical records (EMR) or other information technology functions leading to increased efficiency.

- *Overhead.* Reimbursement for physician services generally is relatively flat compared to the rising cost of doing business that doctors face. Low overhead is another sign of the efficiency physicians look for in a practice. We discussed in the first chapter of this book that physicians do not move for a new title or to step up the corporate ladder. What they seek is a satisfying work environment where they can focus on patient care and not be constantly distracted by reimbursement, regulatory issues and other hassles.

Following is a graph from Merritt, Hawkins & Associates' 2007 Survey of Primary Care Physicians, in which we asked primary care physicians (family practitioners, general internists, and pediatricians) to quantify overhead in their practices:

What does overhead in your practice currently run as a percent of income?

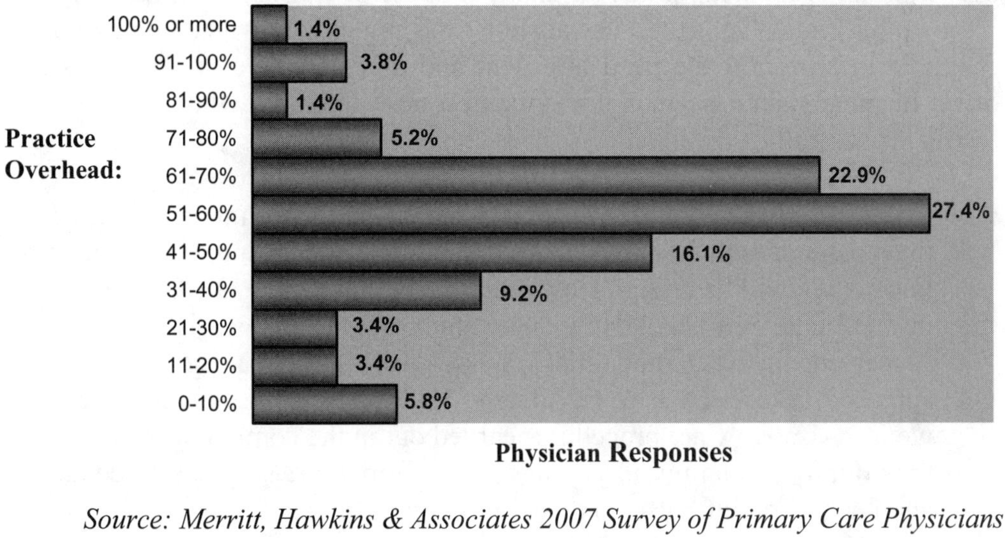

Source: Merritt, Hawkins & Associates 2007 Survey of Primary Care Physicians

As the graph shows, over 60% of primary care physicians said overhead in their practices was 51% or more. The survey also indicated that many primary care physicians are worried about their ability to sustain overhead in their practices, as the following numbers indicate.

Projecting over the next five years, will you be able to support overhead in your practice?

Yes	31.5%
No	13.6%
Doubtful	22.2%
Hopeful	32.7%
N/A	12.0%

Source: Merritt, Hawkins & Associates 2007 Survey of Primary Care Physicians

Low overhead can be one of the key advantages rural hospitals and medical groups can bring to bear in physician recruiting. Rent, labor, and other costs often are less expensive in smaller communities, a fact that can pique the interest of potential candidates in larger communities. Any primary care practice that can boast overhead of less than 50% should do so aggressively. A specialty group with overhead of 40% or less also has a strong selling point to use. By contrast, recruiters representing practice opportunities with relatively high overhead should be able to explain why overhead is high, what is being done to address it, and why even with a relatively high overhead the financial potential in the practice might still be favorable. Even when high overhead limits financial potential, many practice settings are still recruitable if they offer things like generous vacation time, a good call schedule or a very desirable location. If the need is urgent and other positive factors can not offset financial restraints, then it may be necessary to employ the physician to recruit successfully.

- *Type and number of procedures/surgeries.* In addition to knowing who their patients will be, physician candidates want to know the types of things they will be doing. How many deliveries can an OB/GYN expect in the course of a year? How many studies will a radiologist be reading a year and in what modalities? What level of trauma will orthopedic surgeons be expected to see, if any; how much spine, hand or sports work? Also, how are procedures carved out in the community? Is there opportunity for family physicians to perform some surgical procedures and for general internists to do colonoscopies?

- *Nursing/allied staff.* To some extent, physician and nurse staffing go hand-in-hand. One of the principal reasons for physician dissatisfaction is an inadequate nursing staff at the hospital or hospitals with which they are affiliated. This often increases the amount of time they must spend rounding on patients in the hospital and causes patients to complain about poor service. In addition, hospital errors and increased mortality rates have been tied to low nurse to patient ratios and physicians are naturally reluctant to expose their patients to unsafe environments. A particular source of angst among physicians is delayed or limited surgery times due to lack of nurses. One of the first things physicians attempt to do when building specialty hospitals is to recruit all the top nurses in the community so they don't have to deal with these problems.

Again, physicians are primarily concerned about the efficiency of the hospital environment, and this extends to allied health care professionals. A full complement of imaging technologists and lab technologists means two things to physicians: faster scheduling of tests for patients and faster turnaround on the results they need to make timely treatment decisions. It is a significant bonus if recruiters can tout lower than average vacancy rates at the hospital for nurses and allied health professionals.

The numbers below indicate current hospital vacancy rates for several types of health professionals:

Who's Missing?

Hospital Vacancy Rates for Selected Personnel

Registered nurses	8.5%
Nursing assistants	7.6%
LPNs	7.3%
Laboratory technicians	6.3%
Imaging technicians	5.9%
Pharmacists	4.4%

Source: 2006 American Hospital Association Survey of Hospital Leader.

If vacancy rates at your hospital are comparatively low, this is a benefit that should be touted to physician candidates.

- *Who will their colleagues be?* Members of the current medical staff can be a key resource for physician recruiters. Recruiters need to know something about the physicians who are already in the community before they can attract new doctors. These are the people who will help sell the opportunity for you. The best ally of any salesperson is a customer who has bought a product or service and is satisfied with it. Similarly, the best ally of a recruiter is an established doctor who is happy in his or her practice.

Recruiters need to know who the current physicians in the community are – where they went to medical school, where they did their residencies, their board certification status, specialty association memberships, publication record, years in the community, etc. They also need to know the number and types of procedures the physicians perform, the hours they maintain, the incomes they are earning, and the lifestyle amenities they enjoy.

One of the most powerful tools in a physician recruiter's kit is a positive statement about a current physician's practice, such as: "Dr. Smith, you will be joining Dr. Jones. Dr. Jones is board certified in family practice and has been in the community 12 years. Like you, he did his residency at State University Medical Center, and he also has two teenage sons. He currently sees 80 patients a week, is home by 6 p.m. almost every night, and nets $175,000 a year. He keeps horses on his ten acres and his family enjoys their cabin by the lake."

Even if an incoming candidate will have little direct interaction with some members of the medical staff, physicians are very conscious of their peers and want to be assured of the quality and reputation of other doctors with whom they will be associated. Know the staff and be able to explain why a new candidate would be proud to join them.

♦ *Politics.* Of course, not all physicians in the community are going to be positive examples or allies. Those threatened by or otherwise unsupportive of a new physician can easily ruin any chance for success. It is just as important to know about them, so you can deal with the situation on the front end.

Medical politics are much easier to deal with before that moment during a candidate interview when a local doctor unexpectedly announces over lunch that he does not support the search and will do what he can to see that any new doctor fails. While outward displays of this type in a group setting may not happen very often, it is quite common for an unsupportive local physician to express these types of feelings in individual meetings or by telephone after the interview has concluded. An objective opportunity analysis, combined with written and personal staff surveys, can help determine which physicians, if any, are potential road blocks. The analysis should always include face-to-face meetings between the recruiter and any local physicians who are likely to be affected by the search in any way. This should lead to a more accurate understanding about the search and who will be supportive.

These details should be pointed out to potential candidates on the front end. "Dr. Smith, you are going to be meeting Dr. Jones. Dr. Jones is an internist who sees about ten to twelve patients during each of his three half-day clinics per week. He's going to tell you that there isn't enough work for you here, but he could be much busier. He refuses to schedule any additional clinics although the other two local internists, Drs. Rand and Gault, stay very busy seeing twenty-five to thirty patients in each of their four full-day weekly clinics. Non-emergent patients in the area seeking an internist have to wait an average of three weeks for a local appointment. Dr. Jones is happy with his clinic schedule, 1:3 call and his current income. He is not anxious for new competition, regardless of the community's need. However, Dr. Smith, everyone here, from physicians to nurses to administration to local citizens, is supportive of this search effort and anxious to have an additional internist." Providing an explanation for medical politics is the best way to defuse them.

- *Hours/call coverage*. One of the reddest of red flags to watch for in a physician search is a vague or unstated position on what the hours and call coverage situation will be for an incoming physician. "We'll arrange all that when the new doctor gets here" is a statement no physician recruiter should want to hear from a hospital or group administrator. In making a match, you are dealing in expectations and you must lay out precisely what the expectations of both parties are. If the doctors in a group all work 60 hours a week, that expectation should be established on the front end of the conversation with candidates.

- *Incentives/contracts*. Incentives obviously play a vital role in physician recruitment, and Chapter 11 is devoted to the subject of creating a competitive incentive package. The key point we wish to stress here has to do with the physician contract. Whether the new physician is joining an established medical group, will be employed by the hospital, or will set up a solo practice with a hospital's assistance, a contract will be involved. ***It is imperative that a sample contract be prepared and available prior to any in-depth conversations or interviews with candidates.*** No meaningful discussions can take place unless physicians have at least a general idea regarding the terms of the agreement they may be getting into. We have seen many searches delayed or derailed altogether because the recruiting contract is "tied up at corporate" or otherwise unavailable. We liken this circumstance to a wedding that has been meticulously planned but which is ruined at the last moment because the groom has failed to secure a ring, or to a realtor who claims to have a full offer on the table for your house but says he needs a few days to get the contract together.

♦ *Non-competes.* As we mentioned in Chapter Six, when a hospital helps an established medical group to recruit physicians with financial assistance, the group may impose a non-compete on the new physician if non-compete agreements are permissible in the state and if the agreement is structured according to state law. The terms of the non-compete should be delineated in writing in advance of any candidate interviews and subsequently shared with physician candidates who may be interested in the practice.

♦ *Path to partner.* Similarly, there should be no ambiguity about path-to-partner in an existing medical group. Many physicians who end up leaving a practice do so because they believe the path to partnership was not clearly explained to them, or that the established partners did not hold to the terms. "We'll work all that out when you get here" is not a phrase candidates like to hear, because they know it means trouble sooner or later. The key is to work out all of the details on the front end and not wait until they become points of contention on the back end. Keep in mind that in today's market, the concept of "blue sky" is rapidly fading. Partnership buy-ins today are generally based on tangible assets. In some specialties where physicians are in particularly short supply, buy-ins are nominal or even non-existent. We have had radiology and other groups offer full partnership to candidates from day one.

♦ *ER coverage.* In the past, many physicians embraced ER coverage as a method for treating new patients and thereby building their practices. In an era of physician shortages, most physicians don't need to build a practice this way and for a variety of reasons are not enthusiastic about covering the ER. One way hospitals are addressing this challenge is by employing physicians. Others are paying physicians to be on call (see the breakdown of ER coverage pay scales in Chapter 4.)

It is clearly an advantage today not to require ER coverage of new physician recruits, but if that is not feasible, the terms of the coverage arrangement should be spelled out on the front end.

- *Malpractice.* Malpractice rates vary by state and can even vary dramatically within states. Malpractice rates can be a major consideration for physician candidates and studies have shown that the number of physicians applying for medical licenses increases in those states where tort reform has been enacted. If your opportunity is in a state with favorable rates, this advantage should be leveraged in all recruiting communications, including on the hospital or group's web site, in recruiting advertisements, direct mail, etc. If your opportunity is in an area with high malpractice rates, you cannot and should not disguise the fact. However, be prepared to address how other factors such a favorable payer mix, low overhead, and abundant patients may offset the high cost of malpractice insurance. As with opportunities featuring high overhead, it may be necessary to employ the physician and pay for his or her malpractice insurance to recruit successfully.

- *Hospital support.* Some hospitals develop the reputation among doctors for being "physician friendly." Others develop a less positive reputation among physicians. Word within a state and within various specialties travels fast and it is a major recruiting advantage to cultivate a positive reputation. Promoting positive physician relations was discussed in Chapter 4 and we won't repeat ourselves here. Simply keep in mind that you should be able to catalogue the ways in which the hospital provides a good atmosphere for doctors, including things like streamlined patient admission procedures, quick turnaround of patient data, easy parking access, open door administration, updated equipment, a hospitalist program, good nurse-to-patient ratios and access to operating rooms.

A comprehensive opportunity evaluation should provide whoever is acting as the lead recruiter (whether an in-house person or an outside consultant) with all the data they need to paint a picture for candidates of what a day in your opportunity will be like. They should be able to tell the physician what time they will be at work, when they will leave, number of patients they will see, who those patients are likely to be, types of procedures available, equipment at their disposal, overhead and collection rate in the practice, payer mix, politics, malpractice rates, ER coverage, OR access, path-to-partner, terms of the contract, expected immediate and long-term income in the practice and all the other details doctors want to know when they are considering an opportunity.

Know How to "Talk Doctor"

Having detailed knowledge about the practice is central to a recruiter's ability to "talk doctor" -- that is, to speak with the same vocabulary physicians use and to understand their perspective. Consider your experience with salespeople – particularly those selling high end items such as automobiles and medical equipment. The credible ones are those who know their products inside out. They may not be the most charismatic or the best looking, but they can explain what their product is all about and how it can benefit you, the buyer.

A practice opportunity is less tangible than a car or other product. Even more information is therefore needed to make it "feel" tangible and to allow physician candidates to "get their arms around it." Physicians are particularly swayed by data and prefer to hear facts rather than generalities.

A detailed practice analysis, committed to writing, is a fundamental part of the recruiting "iceberg." After all, before you go to the market, you have to know what you are selling.

Examining the Community

An important first step when evaluating your community from the physician candidate's perspective is to remember that almost everyone has geographic biases. Name a state and a certain percentage of physicians will tell you that they would never live there. But that never stopped a good recruiter, and there are thousands of physicians now practicing in places where they never thought they would set foot.

There is nothing you can do about where your community is located. Short of a shift in tectonic plates, where you are is pretty much where you are. In examining your community, however, you can look for those things that tend to refute the prejudices doctors are likely to have and that will convince them that they really can enjoy the type of lifestyle they are seeking in your community. In addition, emphasize those details that may set your community apart. "A friendly town with nice people and good schools" is a generalization that should be supported with facts, including local employment statistics, student-to-teacher ratios, cost of living comparisons, and other details that support a positive portrayal of the area. Don't let emotions about your community get in the way of your objectivity – listen to what candidates are saying, even if the comments are not always flattering, and make adjustments to your approach if necessary.

Here are a few places to start:

- *Current physician lifestyles.* Location is all about lifestyle, and you should be prepared to illustrate the type of lifestyles physicians now located in your community enjoy. What is interesting or appealing about the lifestyles of your physicians? Can they afford second homes or condos at the beach or in the mountains? Do they have homes on multi-acreage? Do they raise horses or keep a small plane at the local airport? Do they have the option of private schools but choose to send their children to local public schools instead? Are their homes just minutes from the hospital or the office? Are they able to attend all their children's baseball games and recitals? What is it about the community that keeps the physicians who now practice there secure and happy?

- *Real estate.* No discussion with a physician candidate is going very far if the candidate gets the sense that he or she simply has no viable real estate options in your community. It therefore is important to establish current real estate options so that candidates get a clear sense of what is available. Smaller communities that often are at a geographic disadvantage when it comes to physician recruitment usually have an advantage when it comes to real estate. A five bedroom, 3,500 square foot home on an acre that sells for less than $300,000 is going to cause some physicians who think they have to live in a major city to reconsider. If your opportunity is located in an area with high real estate prices, you will need to emphasize resale value, equity-building opportunities and access to the amenities usually available in areas where real estate is expensive.

- *Schools.* Be prepared to support the quality of local schools with data such as percentage of graduates going on to college, student-to-teacher ratios, special programs for advanced students, areas of athletic, musical or other excellence, etc. It is a good idea to have a few "case studies" in mind – students who have gone to the local schools and subsequently achieved distinction at Ivy League colleges or at other prominent universities.

Emphasize that physicians in the community send their children to the public schools, if that is the case. If not, emphasize the private school options.

- *Recreational/cultural amenities.* An effort should be made to personalize all aspects of your community, including the recreational and cultural amenities available. For example, in representing a community in North Dakota, our firm was careful to emphasize that Jack Nicklaus regularly hunted there during quail season. We received numerous inquiries from physicians asking about "that community where Jack Nicklaus hunts." We also will make sure to specify in recruiting letters and other candidate sourcing materials some particulars when it comes to entertainment and culture. Indicating that Reba McIntyre recently played at the local concert hall and that the touring Broadway production of "The Producers" recently played at the local theater says a lot more about options in the community than the general statement "we have a lot of culture to offer here." Because physicians hear about so many opportunities, it is these details that allow them to separate one community from another. Again, tying recreational and cultural options back to the lifestyle of physicians already in the community is key. The fact that Dr. Smith maintains a cabin in the mountains or that Dr. Jones has a houseboat on the lake paints a vivid picture of the lifestyle available. Anything that sets your community apart in a positive manner is an advantage.

- *The Internet.* Keep in mind that most communities have a Chamber of Commerce and most Chambers maintain a web site about the communities they represent. Make sure that both your hospital or group web site and the Chamber of Commerce site in your community are putting out a positive message to physicians. Choose pictures of the community wisely and work with the Chamber to include a section about health care delivery in the community and why health professionals enjoy living and working there. Consistency also is important. Make sure whatever you say in recruiting letters and other messages is consistent with what is on the Chamber web site and other sources of information about the community.

Almost every community has positives and negatives. San Francisco is a beautiful city, but it is expensive to live there. Baxter, Iowa provides a terrific family location but it is a long way from the mountains or the ocean. The key in presenting your community and practice opportunity to physicians is to control the flow of information so that doctors don't rule out the community before they have had a chance to truly evaluate it. There is a definite art to this part of the recruiting process, which is discussed in more detail in Chapter 14.

CHAPTER 10

CANDIDATE PARAMETERS

After making a thorough analysis of your practice opportunity and community, you are ready to specify the type of physician you are looking for. Just as we ask physicians to separate what they *want* in a practice from what they really *need,* we counsel hospitals, medical groups and other health care organizations to look for what they really need in a physician instead of insisting on candidates who fit an idealized mold.

Of course, hospitals and other health care organizations want their medical staffs to shine, so the temptation is there to insist on "Dr. McDreamy" – for example, an Ivy League trained physician who looks like he just wandered in from Central Casting.

These types of candidates bear little resemblance to the rapidly changing demographic make-up of physicians today. For one thing, a young physician today is just as likely to be a woman as a man. In some specialties a young doctor may be *more likely* to be a woman, as the numbers below indicate:

Percentage of Medical Residents Who are Female

OB/GYN	68%
Pediatrics	65%
Dermatology	54%
Psychiatry	49%
Family Practice	47%
Pathology	47%
Internal Medicine	40%

Source: Association of American Medical Colleges

In addition, many hospitals and medical groups prefer their physician candidates to be young, generally under 50 and even under 45. Often, this is because they prefer a doctor who is willing to stay a long time in their community, not one who may soon retire. Discriminating against older candidates, however, is impractical and may be illegal. Consider that 33% of all physicians (or over 240,000 doctors) are 55 years old or older. As the following table indicates, physicians in some specialties are older than others:

Medical Specialties by Age

Specialty	% 46 and older	% 56 and older
Psychiatry	71%	43%
Urology	65%	41%
Orthopedic Surgery	61%	35%
Otolaryngology	59%	34%
Family Practice	52%	22%
Internal Medicine	48%	21%

Source: AMA Physician Masterfile

In some specialties, if hospitals or groups were to rule out doctors over 45 they are left with less than half the total potential candidates to choose from. If 55 is the cut-off number, the candidate pool is reduced by over 40% in some cases. While it is true that some older physicians may be near retirement and are not long-term prospects, there are many doctors in their fifties or older who plan to practice for years to come. Others may only practice for a handful of years, but can still be valuable contributors to health care delivery during that time -- and they will certainly be an improvement over *no physician at all.*

The fact is, in today's market, most hospitals and other organizations will simply not succeed if they don't consider the entire range of potential candidates.

The concept is illustrated in the next chart. The figures show the total number of orthopedic surgeons in the U.S. Consider what would happen if a hospital insisted on narrow parameters and would not consider those physicians who are non-board certified, who are 55 or older or who are international medical graduates. Then consider that they could only choose from the number of doctors who change practices each year (9% according to an American Medical Group Association survey on physician turnover). Of these, let us suppose that candidates could be distributed evenly across all 50 states. In a given year, how many orthopedic surgeons would be available per state?

How Many Orthopedic Surgeons?

Total orthopedic surgeons in patient care ...	18,769
Less non-board certified	13,513
Less 55 and older	8,783
Less international medical graduates	7,992
9% who move per year	719
Divided by 50 for each state	14
Total available per state	**14**

Fourteen orthopedic surgery candidates may seem sufficient for Montana or other states with small populations, but 14 is a woefully inadequate number for a state like California, which has hundreds of openings for orthopedic surgeons.

Of course, physicians do not gravitate to all states equally, and the table above is just a theoretical illustration that does not purport to show how many orthopedic surgery candidates really are available per state, per year. What it does show, however, is how quickly the candidate pool shrinks if you insist on narrow parameters. The situation is more dire if you happen to be in one of those states not generally preferred by physicians seeking practice relocation (see the chart below).

States Preferred by Physicians Seeking Relocation:

48% prefer six states

Texas, Florida, North Carolina, New York, California, Washington

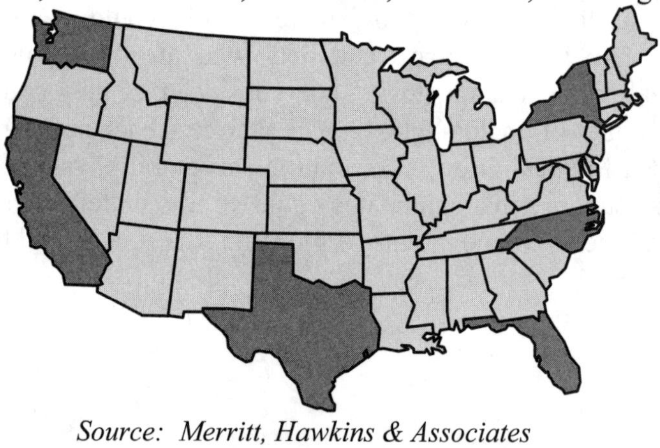

Source: Merritt, Hawkins & Associates

Unfortunately, rural communities are not high on most physicians' wish lists, regardless of what state they are located in. In Merritt, Hawkins & Associates 2006 Survey of Final Year Medical Residents, we asked physicians coming out of training in what type community they would prefer to practice based on population size. Their responses are as follows:

Based on Population, In What Size Community Would You Like to Practice?

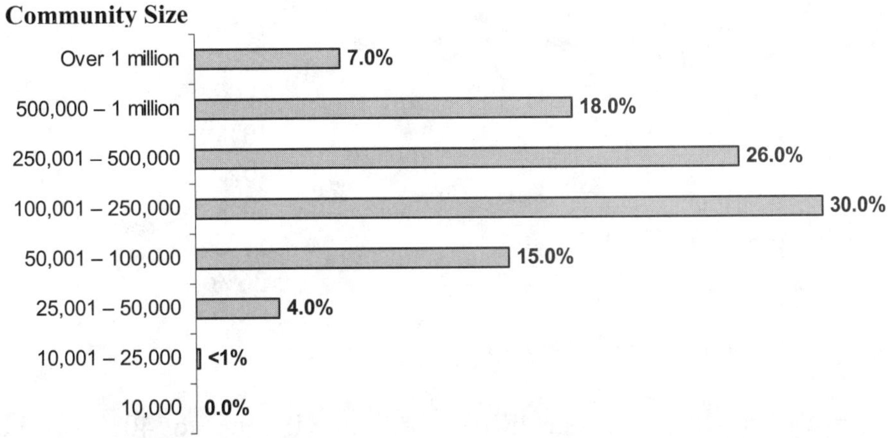

Source: MHA 2006 Survey of Final Year Medical Residents

Of close to 300 new doctors surveyed, only one expressed a preference for practicing in a community of 25,000 or fewer people. This underlines once again the importance of setting candidate parameters that are realistic in the context of today's physician market preferences and demographics.

The demographic question brings us to the subject of international medical graduates, a topic that merits examination in some detail.

A Word About International Medical Graduates (IMGs)

At one time not too long ago, physicians who earned their medical degrees outside of the U.S. were something of an anomaly. When we began recruiting physicians over 20 years ago, many if not most clients simply would not consider IMGs as viable recruiting candidates. Today, such an attitude is no longer realistic and often can be counterproductive. IMGs, by virtue of their sheer numbers and the contributions they are making to health care delivery, have become a resource so indispensable that our health care system would be unable to function without them.

Statistics tell part of the story. One quarter of physicians active in patient care today are IMGs. In some specialties, the percentage is higher, as the numbers below indicate:

International Medical Graduates by Specialty

Specialty	International Medical Graduates
Nephrology	40%
Anesthesiology	32%
Psychiatry	31%
Internal medicine	30%
Cardiology	30%
Neurology	30%
Pulmonology	27%
Gastroenterology	26%

Source: AMA Physician Master File

Administrators who discount IMGs are removing up to 40% of their potential candidate pool right off the top, depending on the type of specialist they are recruiting.

While growing in number, IMGs also are moving from the periphery of the medical establishment to the core. Pick up just about any directory of state or regional medical societies and you will see that IMGs are playing a prominent leadership role in organized medicine. The same holds true for hospital staffs, as IMGs are serving as department heads and medical directors at hospitals throughout the country. At many of the hospitals where we have worked, IMGs are among the top admitters on the medical staff.

In the past, administrators could disregard IMGs and still stand a reasonable chance of filling the majority of their medical staff positions. Market realities today, however, demand an approach to physician staffing that is both free of pre-conceived notions and inclusive of the widest number of appropriate candidates.

The key is to simply apply the same criteria to IMGs as one would to graduates of U.S. medical schools. Training and ability are two critical areas to examine. Just like U.S. graduates, many IMGs are exceptionally well trained, and all have completed U.S. residency programs and the U.S. medical qualifying exam (USMLE or its predecessors.)

Communication and patient rapport also are critical. For the last several years, IMGs have been obliged to pass the Clinical Skills Assessment test, which evaluates their ability to interact with and communicate treatment plans to American patients. Nevertheless, some IMGs still lack sufficient communication skills to be acceptable candidates (but so do some U.S. graduates.)

While training and the ability to communicate are important, a third element is equally critical: desire. The ideal candidate is one who is competent, good with patients, ***and wants to live and practice in your community***. Doctors who fit these parameters are too rare and valuable today not to consider, whether they are tall, short, blue, green, U.S. graduates or IMGs.

Trust Your Patients

In the past, hospital and medical group administrators have told us that they would like to consider IMGs but were concerned that their patients would not accept foreign physicians. That may have been true in the past, but times change. There are hundreds of communities throughout the country – from rural towns to the inner city – where IMGs form the backbone of patient care. Administrators today can trust their patients to accept IMGs provided they demonstrate the qualities referenced above – competence, a warm bedside manner, and the clear desire to serve the community.

It may be true that a particular community has had a poor experience with an IMG who did not demonstrate these traits. However, a bad experience with a U.S. graduate does not preclude most health facilities from ever considering other U.S. graduates, and the same should hold true for IMGs.

Will They Leave?

According to the September 1, 2004 issue of *JAMA,* there are over 6,000 IMGs in U.S. residency programs who are on J or H visas. After they finish training, many of these physicians will need to work in federally designated health professional shortage areas (HPSAs) if they wish to stay in the United States. Once they complete their obligations to work in these areas, some of these physicians will leave for communities they deem to be more desirable.

This is a potential negative to hiring those IMGs who must fulfill visa obligations. However, it should be considered that these obligations can last up to six years. It also should be considered that physicians of all kinds are more mobile today and that there is no assurance that either an IMG or a U.S. graduate is going to stay in any particular community indefinitely.

Whether or not the United States should be so reliant on IMGs is a legitimate question. If, as an industry and as a society, we ultimately decide we should end this reliance, then significant, costly, and time-intensive steps will have to be taken to educate and train more U.S. graduates.

Until then, health leaders should evaluate international medical graduates by the same criteria they use to evaluate their U.S. medical graduate counterparts.

Who Else is Looking?

When deciding what type of physician to seek, it is important to consider who else is looking for physicians today. The answer, of course, is "just about everybody," as the table below suggests.

Hospitals Currently Recruiting Physicians

100 beds or less............75%
101 beds to 200 beds......95%
201 beds or more...........98%

Source: MHA 2005 Survey of Hospital Physician Recruiting Trends

Most hospitals today have at least one person specifically dedicated to recruiting physicians. There are also several hundred physician recruiting firms in the country. Most of them are small, but there are a handful of national firms. Between "in-house" hospital physician recruiters and recruiters working for search firms, there are approximately 6,000 people in the U.S. engaged in physician recruitment. That means one recruiter for every four or so doctors coming out of training each year. That is a lot of people going after the same group of doctors, and it is one reason why new doctors get so many job solicitations (see the following chart.)

How Many Times During Your Training Were You Contacted About Medical Job Opportunities?

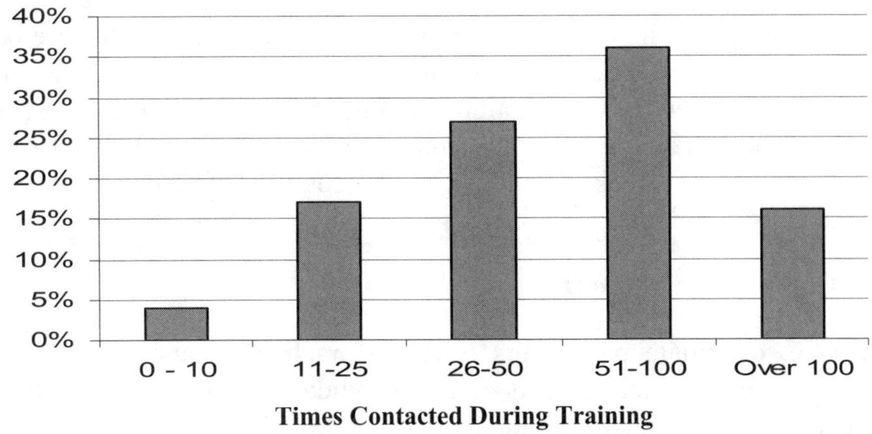

Source: Merritt, Hawkins & Associates 2006 Survey of Final Year Medical Residents

As these numbers show, residents coming out of training have targets on their backs. Everyone knows that at a certain time of year, new doctors will need jobs. Like the very best high school football players who have colleges begging them to sign, residents and fellows have practice options everywhere. For that reason alone, it is a mistake to focus candidate parameters too narrowly on residents or fellows. In addition, residents are not always equipped to make long-term decisions about practice opportunities. Without having much experience with the business of medicine they may not know what they truly need in a practice. This is the main reason why so many physicians coming out of residency leave their initial practice setting after one to two years.

Two Ways to Immediately Improve Your Chances of Recruiting Physicians.

We are frequently asked by clients how they can improve their physician recruiting success. There are two things hospitals, medical groups and other health care organizations can do that will greatly enhance their ability to recruit physicians without costing them a penny.

1: Open the search to older physicians.

2: Seriously consider international medical graduates.

If health care organizations would simply do these two things, they would find their success rate in physician recruitment considerably enhanced.

The principal point, however, is to craft candidate parameters that are both positive and realistic. Focus on the tangible and intangible qualities your patient population needs. Good training, a winning bedside manner, a strong work ethic, and the ***desire to be in your community*** trump an Ivy League pedigree, movie star looks, youth, gender, country of origin and other peripheral considerations.

Avoid "Comparison Shopping"

Of course, candidate parameters have no practical meaning unless you adhere to them. Once agreed upon, candidate parameters should be committed to writing and all stakeholders in the recruiting process must agree that ***an offer will be made to the first physician who meets the predefined requirements.***

This last step is essential to avoid the "comparison shopping" that derails so many physician search efforts. Having interviewed one physician, it is tempting to interview others to see if you can find a candidate who is just that much more qualified or appealing. In today's market that is an error, because while you are looking at candidate two, candidate one is being pursued by other hospitals or medical groups and may not be available should you decide that the grass is not really greener on the other side. Like the fellow who keeps several young ladies guessing as to whom he will ask to the prom (and ends up lonely on Prom Night), you are likely to end up with no one if you are not decisive.

CHAPTER 11

THE INCENTIVE PACKAGE

Before a hospital or medical group begins the process of sourcing potential physician candidates, it should determine what incentives it is prepared to offer. A first step is to consider the purpose of the physician recruiting incentive package.

The principal purpose of the incentive package is to demonstrate to candidates the basic viability of the practice opportunity. Recruiting incentives are essentially the security the recruiting party is putting up to convince physicians that the opportunity is viable.

It is important to consider that for most physicians ***fear of loss outweighs the potential for gain.*** The incentive package allays the fear of loss physicians may incur in relocating to an opportunity, while demonstrating the seriousness of purpose of the recruiting party. It is a starting point that confirms that a real practice is available with real patients. Once this is established, the conversation can progress to what physicians generally are really looking for: ***Quality of life and quality of practice.***

With few exceptions, physicians today are not "chasing a dollar." In today's market, however, dollars often are chasing them. Physicians are hearing from recruiters from all over the country, they have access to a growing number of physician compensation surveys, and they usually have a pretty good idea of what their value is in the marketplace. Incentives must be at a certain competitive level simply to get the conversation going.

A competitive incentive package will typically not be enough to persuade a physician to sign a contract – but competitive incentives are essential in order to get physicians to at least consider an opportunity. The great majority of potential physician candidates are already in practice somewhere else. Physician recruiters have the difficult task of persuading doctors to abandon what they have for something they may ***potentially*** gain.

Keep in mind that recruiting contracts are typically temporary in nature, usually lasting one to two years. After this initial period, during which the physician is generally guaranteed a certain level of income, doctors must sink or swim on their own, unless they are directly employed on a salary. While it may not seem like the physician is taking a big risk, look at it this way.

Suppose a hospital CEO was paid a guaranteed income for one year, and then was paid strictly based on the hospital's performance going forward? A CEO would have to be awfully confident about the hospital's potential performance before agreeing to such an arrangement.

Without a competitive incentive package, physicians are essentially operating without a net – trusting that they will be able to come to a new community and build a practice at least as good as the one they may have left.

In a word, incentive packages are all about ***credibility.***

Tailoring the Package

One size does not necessarily fit all when it comes to physician recruiting incentive packages. The financial package will be shaped and influenced by a number of interacting factors, as illustrated in the "recruiting incentive molecule" below.

The Physician Recruiting Incentive "Molecule"

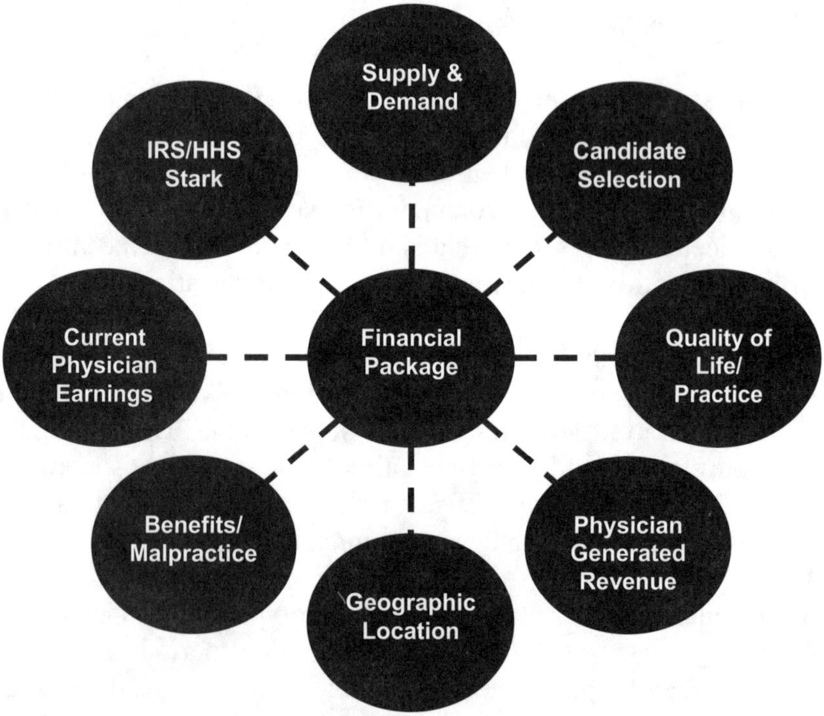
Supply & Demand
IRS/HHS Stark
Candidate Selection
Current Physician Earnings
Financial Package
Quality of Life/ Practice
Benefits/ Malpractice
Physician Generated Revenue
Geographic Location

Each part of the molecule may affect the incentive package. For example, a limited supply of physicians in a particular specialty coupled with an acute demand obviously will drive income offers upward. Conversely, a widely desired geographic location may have a modifying effect on the salary or income guarantee being offered. A practice in a resort area or a popular city typically will offer less than a practice in an area that is not widely perceived to be desirable – even though the "popular" location has a higher cost of living than the unpopular one. This is in part because more candidates generally are interested in the "popular" locations, which, to some extent, are seller's markets (though seller's markets in physician recruitment are rare today.). Additionally, reimbursement rates in popular coastal areas in the West and Northeast often are not as robust as they are in the Midwest or the Southeast, while competition may be greater. This reduces physician incomes and may affect the financial offer.

As discussed earlier, federal physician recruiting regulations require that financial offers be "reasonable" within the context of the specialty being recruited, the geographic area, and the community need for a new physician, and this may put limitations on the offer. If the practice does not offer the physician much personal time, then the financial and benefits package may have to be adjusted upward.

While being competitive is important, you also must be realistic. As discussed earlier, a medical staff plan and a thorough practice analysis will allow a hospital or group to assess the realistic financial potential of the practice. If the staff plan shows a high level of patient migration in a particular service line, a relatively low physician to population ratio, long wait times for appointments and other factors demonstrating that a new physician is needed, then the financial potential in the practice is likely to be high. This will allow for an incentive package in the upper range of the specialty.

Whatever financial incentive is offered should be based on an objective assessment of the practice environment. In a case where a hospital is recruiting into an existing group, the incomes of the established physicians should be a clear indication of the financial potential in the practice, unless there are other circumstances driving incomes down, such as physicians slowing down as they near retirement. The incentive package should not set physician candidates up for disappointment by providing them with an income that is higher than they will realistically be able to make once they are paid solely on their own production, as is eventually the case in most groups. This is a proven way to ensure a high rate of physician turnover in the community.

As mentioned already, there are circumstances when employment is necessary to recruit, sometimes with a salary that exceeds the true short and long-term potential of the practice due to high malpractice rates or reimbursement issues. In these cases long-term employment may be required to avoid physician turnover.

Physician Compensation Data

A number of physician compensation surveys are available that track physician incomes by specialty. The numbers below are derived from <u>Modern Healthcare</u> magazine's 2007 review of physician compensation surveys.

Anesthesiology

Medical Group Management Association (MGMA)	$372,820
American Medical Group Association (AMGA)	$357,430
Merritt, Hawkins & Associates	$300,000
Sullivan, Cotter & Associates	$352,690
Hospital & Healthcare Compensation Services (HHCS)	$320,146
Hay Group	$328,000

Cardiology (non-invasive)

Medical Group Management Association (MGMA)	$394,240
American Medical Group Association (AMGA)	$428,222
Hospital & Healthcare Compensation Services (HHCS)	$291,131
Merritt, Hawkins & Associates	$391,000
Sullivan, Cotter & Associates	$400,428
Hay Group	$347,800

Emergency medicine

Medical Group Management Association (MGMA)	$257,409
Merritt, Hawkins & Associates	$239,000
Sullivan, Cotter & Associates	$248,457
American Medical Group Association (AMGA)	$258,211
Hay Group	$207,600
Hospital & Healthcare Compensation Services (HHCS)	$240,399

Family Practice

Medical Group Management Association (MGMA)	$173,670
Hospital & Healthcare Compensation Services (HHCS)	$156,673
American Medical Group Association (AMGA)	$195,341
Sullivan, Cotter & Associates	$179,576
Hay Group	$165,500
Merritt, Hawkins & Associates	$161,000

General Surgery

American Medical Group Association (AMGA)	$346,996
Medical Group Management Association (MGMA)	$327,867
Hospital & Healthcare Compensation Services (HHCS)	$339,341
Merritt, Hawkins & Associates	$301,000
Hay Group	$268,300
Sullivan, Cotter & Associates	$312,036

Internal Medicine

Medical Group Management Association (MGMA)	$188,270
Hay Group	$173,900
Hospital & Healthcare Compensation Services (HHCS)	$193,471
American Medical Group Association (AMGA)	$199,202
Sullivan, Cotter & Associates	$181,050
Merritt, Hawkins & Associates	$174,000

Neurology

Hospital & Healthcare Compensation Services (HHCS)	$198,312
Medical Group Management Association (MGMA)	$259,867
American Medical Group Association (AMGA)	$237,140
Merritt, Hawkins & Associates	$234,000
Sullivan, Cotter & Associates	$231,496
Hay Group	$209,200

OB/GYN

Medical Group Management Association (MGMA)	$292,569
American Medical Group Association (AMGA)	$297,592
Merritt, Hawkins & Associates	$247,000
Hospital & Healthcare Compensation Services (HHCS)	$243,896
Hay Group	$247,500
Sullivan, Cotter & Associates	$253,646

Oncology

Merritt, Hawkins & Associates	$339,000
Sullivan, Cotter & Associates	$307,903
American Medical Group Association (AMGA)	$345,729
Hospital & Healthcare Compensation Services (HHCS)	$278,028
Hay Group	$351,600
Medical Group Management Association (MGMA)	$492,925

Pathology

Medical Group Management Association (MGMA)	N/A
Sullivan, Cotter & Associates	$280,767
American Medical Group Association (AMGA)	$310,931
Hospital & Healthcare Compensation Services (HHCS)	$200,514
Hay Group	$227,400
Merritt, Hawkins & Associates	$255,000

Pediatrics

Medical Group Management Association (MGMA)	$184,809
Hay Group	$161,800
American Medical Group Association (AMGA)	$197,460
Hospital & Healthcare Compensation Services (HHCS)	$174,077
Sullivan, Cotter & Associates	$175,091
Merritt, Hawkins & Associates	$159,000

Psychiatry

Medical Group Management Association (MGMA)	$203,142
Merritt, Hawkins & Associates	$186,000
Hay Group	$183,200
American Medical Group Association (AMGA)	$209,778
Sullivan, Cotter & Associates	$180,914
Hospital & Healthcare Compensation Services (HHCS)	$177,334

Radiology

Medical Group Management Association (MGMA)	$453,598
American Medical Group Association (AMGA)	$433,253
Hospital & Healthcare Compensation Services (HHCS)	$353,038
Merritt, Hawkins & Associates	$380,000
Hay Group	$375,000
Sullivan, Cotter & Associates	$436,104

Urology

Medical Group Management Association (MGMA)	$395,693
American Medical Group Association (AMGA)	$391,238
Hospital & Healthcare Compensation Services (HHCS)	$325,831
Merritt, Hawkins & Associates	$400,000
Sullivan, Cotter & Associates	$337,131
Hay Group	$269,600

By comparing these surveys, recruiters can get a good feel for the general compensation ranges in various specialties.

The data above includes numbers derived from the Review of Physician Recruiting Incentives that Merritt, Hawkins & Associates compiles every year. The Review summarizes the financial and other incentives that our clients offered to physicians in over 3,000 search assignments from March 31, 2006 to April 1, 2007.

A copy of the 2007 Review of Physician Recruitment Incentives is included in this book.

Our review is distinct from other compensation surveys because it shows not what physicians in various specialties make per year, but the average salary or income guarantees being offered to recruit them. The Review also shows other incentives that hospitals and medical groups are using to recruit physicians, including signing bonuses, relocation allowances, CME allowances, educational loan forgiveness and other perks.

Signing bonuses have become an increasingly popular recruiting tool because they can help "tilt the balance" when physicians are considering various opportunities. If two opportunities are equal in most respects, a signing bonus may provide the timely incentive that "closes the deal."

Signing bonuses are now employed by the majority of Merritt, Hawkins & Associates' clients, as the table below from our 2007 Review of Physician Recruiting Incentives illustrates:

Was A Signing Bonus Offered?

Yes.................................72%
No...................................28%

Amount of Bonus?

Low	Average	High
$5,000	$20,000	$100,000

Who Moves for the "Average Offer?"

As we have stated earlier, the great majority of potential physician recruiting candidates are physicians who already are in practice. To persuade them to move, something about the opportunity clearly has to at least have the potential to be better than where they are now. If you offer the "base line" or "average" compensation package, you must ask yourself what type of doctor the "average offer" is likely to attract. Sometimes, it is a physician who considers the base line to be a raise. However, a candidate with a good current practice will often at least consider an opportunity with greater financial potential.

In order to pique the interest of highly qualified candidates it is best to offer a compensation package that is at least somewhat higher than the average. The idea that you can "buy a good physician" is generally an erroneous one, at least in the long-term. But what a competitive compensation package can do is convince a physician that you have an opportunity worth picking up the phone and exploring – which is all that a good recruiter asks.

Determining what incentives you are prepared to offer is part of the process of creating a competitive recruiting environment. Another is crafting a contract that positions you for success in today's market, a subject we pursue in Chapter 12.

CHAPTER 12

PHYSICIAN RECRUITING CONTRACTS: WHEN MORE THAN A HANDSHAKE IS NECESSARY

A physician recruiting contract should be constructed in a way that is favorable and attractive to physician candidates while protecting the core interests of the recruiting party. The contract should be as simple and straightforward as possible so that it does not become a roadblock or a point of contention between the candidate and the recruiting entity. It stipulates clearly, in writing, the type of behaviors the hospital or group expects from the physician and will reward, while also maintaining the rights and interests of the physician recruit.

A standard physician recruiting contract typically will cover a variety of issues, which we address individually below.

Work Status

The contract will stipulate the new physician's work status. Is the physician an employee of the group or hospital, an independent contactor, a shareholder, and/or a partner? As an employee, physicians generally will be paid a salary, often with a bonus based on "productivity." As an independent contractor, physicians usually will be offered an "income guarantee."

Salaries

A salary offers physicians the security of knowing exactly what their minimum earnings will be. With a salary, there is no risk that the physician will fall below a set income level. However, a salary alone also may reduce the physician's incentive to see patients and be productive, since they will be paid at the same rate for seeing 10 patients a day as for seeing 20.

For this reason, the majority of hospitals and groups offer salaries that feature a production bonus. The production bonus allows the physician to earn above the fixed amount and rewards the physician's extra effort.

In a hypothetical example of a production-based bonus, a new physician employee of a single specialty internal medicine group will be provided with a salary of $160,000 per year. The production bonus will allow the physician to keep 50% of all billings or collections after he or she has generated revenue equal to their breakeven (base salary plus their overhead or share of overhead). The sooner the physician reaches this threshold, the sooner he or she can keep 50% of the billings or collections that they generate from that point forward (under some formulas physicians can keep up to 95% of billings or collections.). There should be some expectation conveyed to the physician (though it may not be put in writing) as to what their gross is likely to be when salary and production are combined. This sets the financial potential in the practice and usually is based on the incomes of doctors already in the practice who are successful.

The "50%" model referenced above is fairly standard, though we have seen contracts that allow new physicians to keep up to 100% of their production after generating revenues in excess of their breakeven, or as little as 40%. This is the most basic type of production bonus, but there are a variety of others.

In some contracts, production may be based not just on number of patients seen but on the *type* of patient seen. Not all patients are equal. Again, in the example of the internal medicine group, one physician may be seeing a high percentage of elderly patients with chronic problems. These patients take more time than younger, "well-care" patients. If the new doctor's practice is comprised of mostly older, chronic patients, he or she won't be able to see as many patients as a physician seeing well patients. In a production-based contract that rewards physicians for number of patients seen, the new doctor could be penalized for having an older patient base.

Is it more favorable to the candidate to have a contract where the production bonus is based on billings or on collections? That depends on the patient base in the practice. If the candidate is taking over the practice of a departing physician whose patient base had a strong payer mix, then a production bonus based on collections would be appropriate. However, if the candidate's payer mix is likely to be poor with a high percentage of no pay or low reimbursing patients, then a savvy candidate will seek a production bonus that is based on Relative Value Units (RVUs) so that they are not penalized by the lower collections. Groups hiring a new physician should always funnel as many new patients as possible to the new physician to ensure that he or she is able to build a diverse patient base with a healthy payer mix as soon as possible.

As mentioned above, some contracts base production not on number of patients seen but on the amount of work done by physicians. In these contracts, work is measured by a point system based on RVUs. A physician seeing a high number of older patients will get more points per patient than a physician seeing mostly younger well patients. At the end of the day, the amount of work physicians are doing will be equal and their pay will be equal – at least that is the idea behind these types of contracts.

These contracts also may provide compensation for things other than patient care, such as scores on patient satisfaction surveys, participation in group governance, and on positive outcomes. However, in today's environment, governance and other issues are taking a clear back seat to production.

While there are a variety of ways to "slice the pie" in a medical practice, the one which seems to work best in our experience is the simple one in which new physicians get paid a base salary that is predicated on current physician income data for their specialty supplemented by a bonus based upon production. Again, it is important that the terms are clear in the contract so that the new physicians know what is expected and have a clear path for achieving a certain level of income.

Income Guarantees

The physician contract will be different if the doctor is being recruited as an independent practitioner rather than as an employee. Though medical groups are playing a growing role in physician recruitment, much of the physician recruitment that takes place today is driven by the hospital or hospitals in a given community. Even if the physician is joining a group practice, the group's affiliated hospital may be funding the recruitment and overseeing the recruiting process. It also will be doing so in the case of a solo physician who is coming to the community. The hospital is involved because it wants to ensure quality patient care in its area and ready access to physician services. And, of course, as a byproduct, the hospital also wants to ensure its own financial viability by recruiting physicians who may refer it patients.

Part of the hospital's role in physician recruiting is to provide independent practitioners with an income guarantee. It is the hospital, then, not the group, that is providing physicians with the economic incentive to come to the community. It is the hospital that is taking the economic risk of providing a new physician with money. But the hospital is willing to take this risk because it is confident that a need for a physician exists. The income guarantee is, in fact, the hospital's way of saying it knows there is a need for another physician and is willing to put its money where its mouth is. As mentioned earlier, the hospital will be confident that a need for new physician services exists based on the community physician needs assessment plan it has conducted. The income guarantee, then, serves as an inducement to attract an incoming physician and is a testament to the need for new physician services in the community.

A net income guarantee ensures that the physician will earn a certain amount of income per month, after practice expenses, for a given period of time (typically one to two years). For simplicity's sake, let us say that amount is $20,000 per month, or $240,000 per year.

Each month the physician is guaranteed to receive $20,000 in pre-tax income after expenses are paid. For example, if the physician only generates collections of $10,000 in a given month during the guarantee period, the hospital will pay him or her an additional $10,000 plus expenses. Should the physician's net income (cash collections less all practice expenses) in any month during the guarantee period exceed $20,000, then the physician returns the excess to the hospital until all un-repaid subsidies have been paid or until the guarantee period ends.

After the guarantee period has ended, if the physician has not repaid all subsidies made by the hospital, he or she owes the hospital the un-repaid amount. However, almost all income guarantees include *a forgiveness clause* which comes into play at the end of the guarantee period.

Forgiveness

Under this clause, the hospital agrees to "forgive" any amount the physician may owe at the end of the guarantee period in exchange for the physician's continued service in the area. The period of "forgiveness" generally ranges from one to three years. If, for example, the physician owes the hospital $50,000 in un-repaid subsidies from the guarantee period, that amount will be forgiven on a pro-rated monthly basis over the one to three year forgiveness period.

The physician therefore has an incentive to stay through the entire contract period, which includes the one to two year income guarantee period and the one to three year forgiveness period. Should the physician decide not to stay through the entire contract period, any subsidies still owed to the hospital must be repaid immediately. In addition, any amount of money forgiven by the hospital must be treated by the physician as taxable income.

By this mechanism, the physician is ensured that he or she will earn a certain amount over the guarantee period and will have no financial obligation by staying through the forgiveness period. In effect, the income guarantee is a loan which must be repaid, if not in money then through time spent practicing in the community. Some physicians prefer the relative autonomy of income guarantees, particularly those who have experience and aptitude in the business of medicine. Younger physicians, for the most part, are more comfortable with employment, and many of their more experienced counterparts are beginning to lean that way as well as they seek to reduce administrative hassles and financial risk.

Educational loan forgiveness

Sometimes, hospitals, groups or other employers may agree to reduce newly recruited physician's medical education loans as part of the contract. The Association of American Medical Colleges reports that, on average, graduating medical students are $110,000 in debt, and that 33% of graduating medical students are over $150,000 in debt. With the number of two-doctor families growing, some physicians can easily face a family educational debt of $250,000 or more. Educational debt forgiveness therefore can be a very powerful recruiting incentive. Debt that might burden a physician for years can be reduced in a much quicker time frame through educational loan forgiveness.

The quid pro quo is that the new physician must agree to practice in the community for a certain length of time. The employer might agree to pay the physician's educational debt on a pro rated basis over two or three years. A physician $75,000 in debt therefore would have $25,000 paid off by the hospital per year in exchange for a commitment to stay in the community for three years. If the educational loan is not a federal or state loan, the physician will receive a 1099 form and be required to pay taxes on the amount forgiven.

A contract will be more attractive from the candidate's point of view if the stipulated loan forgiveness amount is paid in full when the candidate starts or at the beginning of each year, not at the end of the three year period. If, for professional or personal reasons, the physician wants or needs to leave the community before three years, he or she will be paid only for the time that they practiced in the community. For example, if the physician leaves after one year, one-third of his or her loans will be paid off. Structured the other way, a new doctor could spend years in the community and have no educational payments to show for it – a risk that will scare off savvy candidates.

Restrictive covenants/non-competes

Some contracts will contain restrictive covenants or non-compete clauses. These clauses oblige new physicians to agree that they will not go to work for specific competitors over a given period of time, or will not set up practice on their own within a certain distance of the community. Usually, the new physician must commit not to practice within a 10, 20, or 30 mile radius of their employer for a certain length of time – typically one to two years. This acts as a barrier to physicians establishing themselves in a community by joining a group and then joining a competing group or setting up shop on their own.

These clauses may not be legal in some states (California is particularly employee friendly when it comes to non-competes.). They are legal in other states as long as they are deemed to be reasonable with regard to both time and distance. As a general rule, a neurosurgeon will be subject to a much wider geographic restriction than a family practitioner. The more specialized the practice – and hence the larger patient population needed to support the practice – the larger the geographic restriction can be.

In Chapter 6, we noted that new Stark regulations released in September, 2007 permit medical groups that have received financial recruiting assistance from a hospital to impose a non-compete clause on new physician recruits if such agreements are permissible in the state. This has caused some groups to be more open to recruiting doctors, since they no longer have to fear that they may be recruiting their future competition.

Hours/duties/call/vacation

One common bone of contention for many newly recruited physicians is hours. Often new physicians enter a group with an expectation that they will work a certain number of hours, only to find that the requirement or common practice in the group is longer hours than they expected. The same holds true for call. Sometimes, it isn't as good as new physicians were led to believe, eventually leading to turnover in the group.

The contract therefore should stipulate the number of hours the new physician will be required to work each week. Today, many contracts acknowledge the desires of Generation X and Y physicians for limited or flexible hours. The contract also should be as specific as possible about the call arrangement. Some contracts are ambiguous, indicating that call will be arranged on an "appropriate" or "fair" basis. It is preferable that call be shared on an equal basis within the group, and that this is laid out in the contract. However, be careful not to commit to a schedule that will later change for the worse. Just as ambiguous contracts can scare candidates away on the front end before they are recruited, candidates will be driven away on the back end after they are recruited if commitments in the contract go unfulfilled.

Outlining duties can be difficult, certainly with regard to productivity, because it is impossible to know in advance how many patients a new physician will see or how many procedures he or she will perform. However, the contract should specify in general what the physician is there to do – what services or procedures, what administrative duties, etc.

Vacation time also should be specified in the contract. Often, this is a negotiating point, and for those specialties in the greatest demand, vacation times are increasing. While 4 or 5 weeks was common in radiology four or five years ago, 8 to 13 weeks is common now. For other specialties such as cardiology and orthopedic surgery, 4 to 8 weeks is common, while in primary care 3 to 6 weeks is standard. However, vacation can fluctuate based on the number of physicians in the practice, culture of the practice and related factors. In addition, almost all contracts include one week off for CME and a CME allowance.

Path to partnership

Path to partnership can be a key negotiating point. In specialties in very high demand, the path to partnership is getting much quicker than the three years that used to be typical. In some cases, new physicians are automatically made partner. In any case, the path should be clear – one year, two years, or three years. Promising a new physician partnership when he or she reaches a "full practice" or when the physician has "met the expectations of the group" is vague and will put off many candidates. Moreover, buy-ins for "goodwill" or accounts receivable in a practice are becoming increasingly rare. Real-estate buy-ins should be an option, not a requirement. Generally, the only buy-ins today require physicians to pay for their share of the depreciated value of the practice's hard assets. A good rule of thumb once you have the right candidate is to make buy-ins as easy as possible.

Benefits

Physicians are similar to other employees today in that they generally are offered benefits which will be spelled out in the contract. Our 2006 Review of Physician Recruiting Incentives (see the back of this book) indicates which benefits are standard today, including to various degrees health insurance, malpractice insurance, disability insurance, retirement and educational loan forgiveness.

Termination

It should be clear under what circumstances a new physician may be terminated. Generally, there are two types of termination provisions: "with cause" and "without cause."

Under the first type, the employer has to provide reasons for which it can terminate a physician. These reasons usually include loss of hospital or prescribing privileges or inappropriate conduct. It is important that these be specific. "Inability to meet patient needs," for example, is a subjective consideration that can be open to wide interpretation.

A "without cause" provision allows the employer to terminate a physician for no stated reason. However, the contract should require that notice be given in writing in advance – usually from 60 to 180 days. This clause applies both ways. Should a physician decide to leave, the required written notice period (which generally is the same length of time for both parties) gives the employer some time to find a replacement. A "without cause" provision should allow the employed physician the option to terminate the contract with no stated reason as long as written notice is given.

A contract is a good thing to have

The contract obviously is the key document in a physician search and, if we can be indulged in an understatement, it is a good idea to have one before you initiate the search. Without such a document, the physician will have a hard time evaluating the practice. With a contract, the entire process can proceed on a firm footing based on clear expectations and clear communication.

This much is clear: time is of the essence. You are running a race with other hospitals and groups to recruit a limited number of physicians. Every race must have a finish line. The contract represents the finish line for securing a physician candidate. A counter-signed contract allows your organization to cross the finish line ahead of all the others who also were chasing your candidate.

CHAPTER 13

CANDIDATE SOURCING

The physician recruiting process now is getting closer to the tip of the "recruiting iceberg." The initial groundwork may have been laborious, but it was necessary to position the recruitment effort for success. Consider what has been achieved so far:

- The recruitment plan is in place
- The plan is compliant with federal regulations
- The stakeholders have been identified
- Channels of communication have been established
- The strengths and weaknesses of the opportunity have been documented
- The terms of the offer are outlined in a sample contract
- Candidate parameters are set in writing

You now are in a position to actively seek candidates.

Where do you look?

Three Candidate Sourcing Principles

The first key sourcing principle to consider is that physician recruiting is not an event, it is a process, and the process never ends. Hospitals and medical groups should be in continual recruitment mode. The first step is to leverage existing contacts, including members of the medical and administrative staff, professional acquaintances, and members of the community. What friends or colleagues do physicians already in the community know who may be interested in practice relocation? Are there students from the community in medical school or residency who may be interested in returning home? Would they accept a yearly stipend in exchange for a commitment to practice in the community?

In addition, many hospitals and groups fail to take full advantage of the residency programs in their areas. Speaking before residents (who are always happy to attend seminars where meals are offered) and developing relationships with residency directors are two fundamental methods of candidate sourcing that should be vigorously pursued. Exhibiting at physician conventions also can be a beneficial way to make personal contact with prospective candidates.

It is important to continually "work" personal contacts, public speaking venues, and media channels to ensure that the word is out that the hospital or medical group is always looking for "a few good men (and women)."

Another key sourcing principle is that you should not rely too heavily on any one particular method of contacting candidates. Instead, consider an "ambient" approach in which candidates see or hear about your recruiting messages from multiple sources, including personal networking, advertising, the Internet, physician conventions and direct mail. Do not expect an avalanche of responses from any one source – quality responses in most specialties rarely amount to more than a handful.

The third principle is what we broadly refer to as "boots on the ground." Regardless of how many ads you run, jobs you post online, or letters you send, at some point someone must get on the phone and talk to candidates. Whether this is an in-house recruiter or an outside firm, someone has to proactively seek out doctors who may be interested in locating to a new opportunity. In today's recruiting market, it is a mistake to believe that physicians will simply come to you if you throw out enough feelers.

This is the point at which a high level of commitment and work ethic are required, because physicians often are not available to speak about relocation during regular working hours. Some of the hard work of calling potential candidates must take place after normal business hours or on weekends. Physician recruiting is similar to executive recruiting in this regard. Most executives are not in a position to speak to recruiters at work, and nor are many doctors.

Before we discuss the "boots on the ground" principle further, however, we will address such candidate sourcing methods as the Internet, advertising and direct mail.

The Internet

In Merritt, Hawkins & Associates' Survey of Final Year Medical Residents, we asked doctors coming out of training how they learned about practice opportunities (see the following chart.)

What Are Your Best Resources for Learning About Medical Practice Opportunities?

Internet 77%
Personal networking 76%
Physician recruiters.........55%
Residency program...........52%
Specialty society..............17%
Journal advertising...........7%

Source: Merritt, Hawkins & Associates' 2006 Survey of Final Year Medical Residents

Clearly, for young doctors, at least, the Internet is an important resource when it comes to researching practice opportunities. An increasing amount of medical education is accomplished online and younger physicians, like younger people in general, are apt to carry on personal and business relationships electronically. Hospitals and medical groups should be set up for such online communication and should maximize their online presence, particularly their web sites.

All hospital and medical group web sites should have a section specifically dedicated to physician recruitment, independent of other employment related information on the site. In the past, if physicians knew little about a community, the recruiter could control the flow of information and strategically prepare the physician for a site visit. Today, a physician can go right to the Internet and research the community, so information is harder to control. It therefore is important that a hospital or medical group's web site present the most appealing portrait possible about the facility and the community.

A key feature to include is ***testimonials from physicians already in the community*** regarding what they like about their practice and the area. Testimonials should cover the physician-friendly aspects of the hospital and particular reasons why the community is right for the physician and his or her family.

The physician recruitment section of the site should mirror in some ways a Chamber of Commerce site, but it should have a doctor orientation. The hospital or group also should monitor the local Chamber site, because physicians are likely to look at it before they agree to interview. The hospital or group's site and the Chamber's site should be consistent in the information they present. This may include real estate information. If real estate values in the community are favorable, it is not a bad idea to include pictures of the types of housing options physicians can enjoy in the neighborhood.

Hospitals and groups should drive traffic to their sites by making sure the site's address is prominent on all recruiting postings, ads, direct mail and other literature.

In addition to getting the most from their own sites, hospitals and groups may wish to post physician practice openings on the large and growing number of physician employment sites on the Internet. Below is a list of some such sites:

Physician Employment Web Sites

- **PracticeLink.com**
- **Gasworks.com**
- **Radworks.com**
- **Radlinks.com**
- **MD Jobsite.com**
- **Healthcareers.com**
- **Practice choice.com**
- **Gasjob.com**
- **Healthcaresource.com**
- **Healthjobusa.com**
- **Doctorwork.com**
- **Practice.org**
- **RADCareers.com**
- **Radworking.com**
- **Radiologyjobs.com**
- **AAFP.org**
- **Healthcarematch.com**
- **ResidencyLists.com**
- **ACPonline.com**
- **Med2020.com**
- **Thedoctorjob.com**
- **Mommd.com**
- **Staffpointe.com**
- **Mojobsite.com**
- **Employmed.com**
- **AllHealthjob.com**
- **HosptialJobsonline.com**
- **Phyjob.com**
- **Ihirephysicians.com**
- **Familyphysiciansjobs.com**
- **Practiceonline.com**
- **Medicalworkers.com**
- **Gastro.org**

It is cost prohibitive for most hospitals or groups to be on more than a select number of sites. Recruiters need to research which sites get the most traffic and reach the most targeted physician audience. They then must keep track of job postings to ensure that they are updated and accurate.

Advertising

Print advertising remains a viable way to source candidates. Many physician publications today also have employment related sites, so that print ads and Internet postings are part of a package deal.

Success in advertising often is a function of frequency, in addition to an effective advertising message. Running just one ad may elicit a satisfactory response, but in general advertising is more effective when it is run over weeks or months. If you consider the way consumers often use advertising you will see why. A need arises – such as the desire to replace worn out tires – and you check the newspaper ads to see which stores are running discounts. Similarly, a physician will have a desire to relocate and will check practice opportunity ads to see what types of positions are available.

Those hospitals and medical groups that maintain a continual presence in medical journals are positioned to attract the notice of those in-practice physicians who at some point have the need or the desire to relocate their practices.

There is another group of candidates that advertising can reach – those who the advertiser knows will have a particular need at a particular time. At the end of every summer, newspapers and magazines are full of ads for school supplies. Stores may run ads for school supplies year-round, because they know that for a minority of consumers the need for school supplies will arise during the school year and they want to capture the interest of those consumers. But they concentrate their advertising at the end of summer when they know the need is at its peak.

In the physician world, graduating residents and fellows represent the "seasonal" consumer who definitely has a need. Budget permitting, we believe this is the best group of physicians to target with advertising, because the great majority of residents at some point in their training are actively seeking jobs, whereas the great majority of in-practice physicians are not. Publications specifically targeted to residents can be an effective advertising vehicle.

"Active" and "Passive" Candidates

One drawback of advertising is that it tends to attract mostly "active" candidates – those physicians who for whatever reason are in need of a job. Typically, this group represents only a fraction of the physician market; in particular, those with training or an obligation of some kind that is about to end. The following graph illustrates this point:

Who's Out There?

"Active" Candidates

	*Residents
	*Military physicians
15%	*Public Health Service Physicians
	*In-practice physicians seeking a job

"Passive" Candidates

85%	*In-practice physicians, not seeking a job but who might move for the right opportunity

In some cases, advertising attracts the "usual suspects," a minority of physicians who for a variety of reasons are regular job seekers. Not all of these doctors may be satisfactory candidates, particularly relative to in-practice physicians who are successful but who are not actively looking.

Again, a principle from the executive recruiting world applies. When a Fortune 500 company needs an executive, the best candidates often are executives who are successfully running companies, not those who are actively looking for a job. While these "passive" candidates are not looking for new employment, they might be persuaded to relocate to another company under the right circumstances. It can be a challenge to reach these candidates through advertising since they are not actively seeking a new position.

By contrast, companies seeking new executives often will target graduating MBAs with advertising, because all MBAs, the strongest candidates and the weakest, at some point will need a job. MBAs and graduating residents are similar in this regard.

The problem with focusing the majority of one's recruiting efforts on residents, however, is that these candidates are so frequently targeted it is hard to break through the clutter. Everyone knows that the 16,000 or so U.S. trained residents who "come out" each year need jobs and everyone tries to recruit them, often to the exclusion of the great majority of physicians who are not looking, but who might be persuaded to do so.

Direct Mail

Internet postings and traditional advertising are two key ways of alerting the physician market to a practice opportunity. A third is direct mail, or what we prefer to call "personal letters."

One advantage of letters personally addressed to physicians is that they reach the "passive" candidates referenced above. While these doctors may not be paying much attention to recruiting ads or visiting job sites, they do open their mail. The entire multi-billion dollar direct mail industry is based on one indisputable fact: ***people do look at their mail.***

According to the experts, consumers will, on average, devote 1.5 seconds in reviewing the contents of direct mail letters. Their eyes go first to the salutation of the letter to see who it is addressed to, then to the close of the letter to see who it is from. If they are interested in the contents, they will read on.

Over the last 20 years, Merritt, Hawkins & Associates has sent tens of millions of personal letters to physicians regarding practice opportunities. These letters have been sent in batches of as few as several hundred to subspecialties with few physicians to as many as 20,000 to specialties with numerous physicians. Each letter describes a particular practice opportunity and is targeted to physicians in a particular specialty.

In addition to reaching passive candidates, personal letters can be highly targeted to reach doctors in specific areas or those doctors with specific levels of training or experience. Through return cards and other mechanisms, response to personal letters can be tracked and it is possible to measure techniques that drive response up, such as the use of an "invitation" format during holiday seasons, a "P.S." at the bottom of the letter and other techniques.

It also is possible in the text of a letter to provide a superior level of detail about a particular opportunity than there may be space for in an Internet listing or print add, including details about practice overhead, payer mix, available procedures, collection rate, income and other matters. Personal letters also provide a useful way of directing physicians to the hospital, group or recruiting company web site.

When researching job opportunities, residents and younger physicians in particular tend to use the Internet. When it comes to being contacted about job opportunities, however, they prefer old fashioned snail mail, according to one survey (see below).

How Do You Prefer To Be Contacted About Job Opportunities?

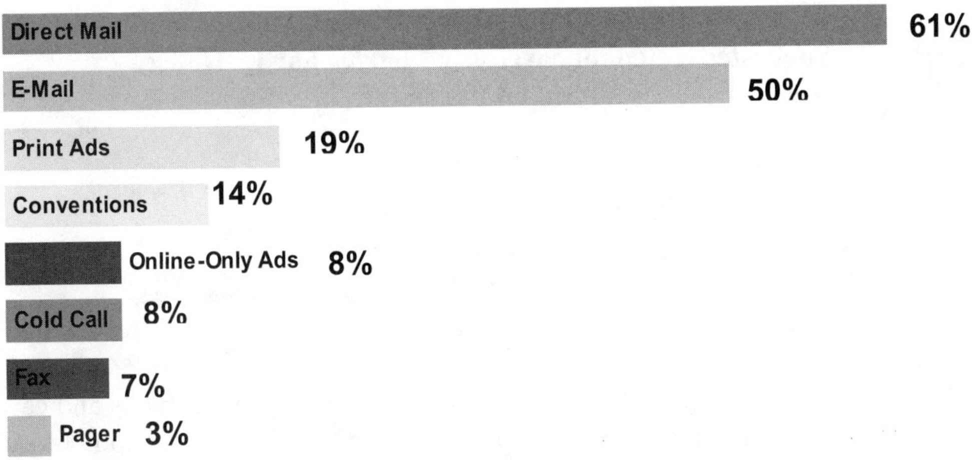

Source: How Young Physicians Search for Jobs, Zeldis Research Associates, April 2004, Conducted for the New England Journal of Medicine

"Boots on the Ground"

A combination of networking, Internet postings, advertising, and direct mail should generate at least some interested candidates. However, in today's market these sourcing methods need to be supported by a proactive effort to contact potential recruits. In essence, what this means is that someone has to pick up the phone and talk to physicians.

Whether the search is being conducted in house or in partnership with a recruiting firm, recruiters trained and adept at speaking to and influencing potential physician candidates must continually "work" the phones to develop pending candidates.

This is part of the "science" of physician recruiting referenced earlier in this book, and it can be boiled down to the following statement:

MEASURABLE ACTIVITY = MEASURABLE RESULTS

Based on two decades of experience, we know that if a well trained recruiter makes a certain number of phone calls to physicians, these calls will lead to a certain number of contacts, which will lead to a certain number of interviews and, ultimately, a certain number of placements.

The table below indicates suggested telephone activity metrics for hospital or medical group in-house physician recruiters:

Suggested Telephone Activity Metrics For In-House Physician Recruiters

- 100 dials per week
- 10 physician contacts per week
- 3 practice opportunity presentations
- 1-2 candidate referrals from physicians contacted
- 1 potential candidate sourced per week

Because in-house physician recruiters often have a variety of duties and can not spend all of their time on the phone, these metrics differ from those Merritt, Hawkins & Associates requires of its recruiters and research consultants.

Our research consultants do nothing but call physicians, and are tasked with making about 100 phone calls a day. Research consultants with Merritt, Hawkins & Associates, including our NewPhysician brand, which targets residents and first and second year doctors, generate over 40,000 phone calls to physicians per month.

Merritt, Hawkins & Associates' recruiting consultants have a variety of duties in addition to making phone calls, and therefore are not tasked with making as many calls as research consultants. Nevertheless, with over 100 recruiters making approximately 60 calls per day, our recruiting consultants generate over 100,000 calls to physicians per month.

On an annual basis, Merritt, Hawkins & Associates generates over 1.5 million calls to physicians per year.

We mention this only partly to "blow our own horn." The principal point, however, is that it takes a defined and measurable level of outreach to identify physician candidates today. You can "cast a net" through job postings, ads, mail and other sources, but someone has to reach out and gather that net in.

Complex as physician recruitment may have become in many ways, the essence is really quite simple: ***You have to talk to doctors!***

Who Are You Going to Call?

No, not "Ghostbusters."

The first physicians to call are those who have been referred by the medical staff or identified through other sourcing methods. Surprising as it may seem, recruiters sometimes let even qualified candidate leads languish due to a natural resistance to picking up the phone and calling a stranger.

It also makes sense to contact those physicians practicing within your state, including residents, and physicians coming out of the military. In specialties with a relatively small number of doctors, geographic location is less of a concern. It is not unusual for Merritt, Hawkins & Associates' recruiters to call through every qualified physician in the country when searching for a sub-specialist.

"Working the phones" is not the easiest task in the world. The fact is that phone calling represents the "nitty gritty" of physician search that few people want to do. Nevertheless, the ***science*** of physician recruiting shows that measurable phone activity is a critical part of the physician recruiting process.

But what do you say to physicians to persuade them to visit your practice opportunity? That's where the ***art*** of physician recruiting comes in, which we discuss in the next chapter.

CHAPTER 14

THE ARC OF PERSUASION

In many cases, physician recruiters are attempting a task that can be considered down right presumptuous.

Often, they are trying to convince a physician that a particular practice opportunity will provide a better professional setting than the physician now is in and that the opportunity will provide a better environment for the physician's family. In essence, recruiters are saying to in practice doctors: "I can make your life better. If you leave your job, leave your house, leave your community, take your kids out of school, you'll be much happier. Trust me." To physicians who are not in practice, such as residents, they are saying: "Put your future career in my hands."

How does a recruiter go from being a stranger on the phone to someone physicians trust so much that they will give up what they have for the better life the recruiter is promising?

There is no magic bullet answer to this question. It comes down to the individual recruiter. Physician recruiters must have a high level of innate sales ability combined with the rigorous training needed to understand the world from the physician's point of view, as well as the various points of view of the people seeking the physician. They also must have the discipline and fortitude to hear the word "no" many times and not be discouraged.

The "Arc of Persuasion"

Given a basic level of ability and training, physician recruiters can take doctors from a level of unfamiliarity and possible distrust, to a point where they are ready to sign a contract, by following what we call the "Arc of Persuasion."

Based on two decades of experience, we know that if a well trained recruiter makes a certain number of phone calls to physicians, these calls will lead to a certain number of contacts, which will lead to a certain number of interviews and, ultimately, a certain number of placements.

The table below indicates suggested telephone activity metrics for hospital or medical group in-house physician recruiters:

Suggested Telephone Activity Metrics For In-House Physician Recruiters

- 100 dials per week
- 10 physician contacts per week
- 3 practice opportunity presentations
- 1-2 candidate referrals from physicians contacted
- 1 potential candidate sourced per week

Because in-house physician recruiters often have a variety of duties and can not spend all of their time on the phone, these metrics differ from those Merritt, Hawkins & Associates requires of its recruiters and research consultants.

Our research consultants do nothing but call physicians, and are tasked with making about 100 phone calls a day. Research consultants with Merritt, Hawkins & Associates, including our NewPhysician brand, which targets residents and first and second year doctors, generate over 40,000 phone calls to physicians per month.

Merritt, Hawkins & Associates' recruiting consultants have a variety of duties in addition to making phone calls, and therefore are not tasked with making as many calls as research consultants. Nevertheless, with over 100 recruiters making approximately 60 calls per day, our recruiting consultants generate over 100,000 calls to physicians per month.

On an annual basis, Merritt, Hawkins & Associates generates over 1.5 million calls to physicians per year.

We mention this only partly to "blow our own horn." The principal point, however, is that it takes a defined and measurable level of outreach to identify physician candidates today. You can "cast a net" through job postings, ads, mail and other sources, but someone has to reach out and gather that net in.

The "Arc" is illustrated below:

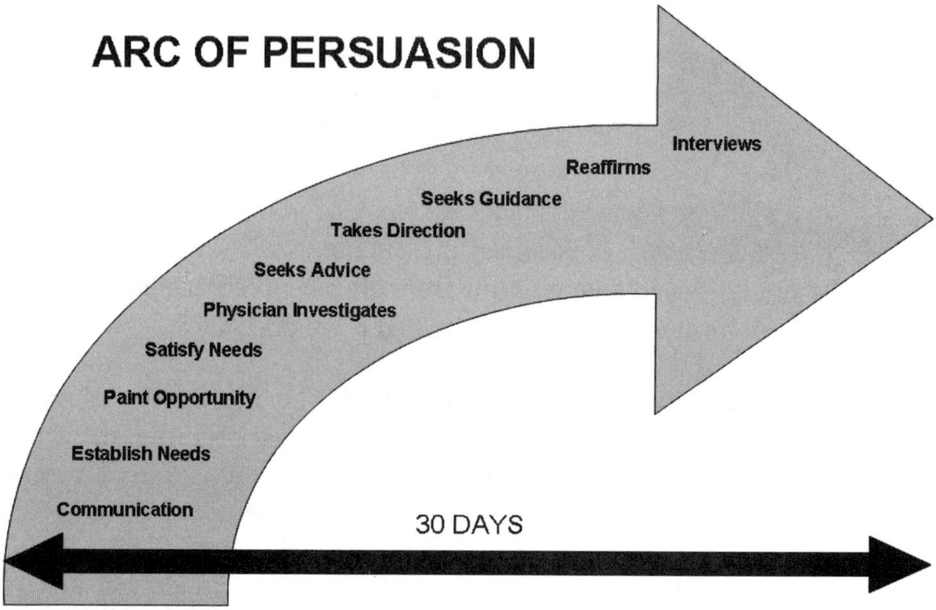

This process often begins before the initial telephone contact has been made. Keep in mind before the first conversation, some physicians may have some knowledge level and respect for your organization. They may have become aware of your hospital or group through a letter or advertisement they have seen, through your web site, or through general word of mouth. If your organization has developed a reputation for being physician-friendly, then half the battle is won before the first telephone contact is made.

However, while name recognition is an important element when a conversation begins, it is not the decisive element. The decisive element is the information the recruiter shares with the physician – both the content of the information and the way it is presented.

The candidate "screen" follows the steps outlined in the "Arc of Persuasion" above. The first task is not to focus on either the professional or personal aspects of the opportunity. Rather, recruiters should make a concerted effort to understand the physician's needs and those of his or her family. Often, physicians will have pre-conceived ideas regarding the geographic location or medical setting they believe they must have to be content. It will only be a rare and happy coincidence if the physician's pre-conceived notion of the ideal location happens to be the community the recruiter represents.

More often than not, recruiters will need to persuade physicians that their opportunity offers the majority of the things the physician needs. This can only be accomplished if the recruiter spends considerable time on the phone with the physician and his or her spouse, learning their needs and aspirations. This is not the way most physicians will want the conversation to start, however. Typically, they will ask, "So, where is this place?" It is at this point that the recruiter must position himself as a consultant, and advise the physician that his or her needs come first, and that before details of the practice can be shared the recruiter must know more about the physician and his or her family. The recruiter then should compile a ***written profile of the candidate*** that describes their motivations, concerns, family situation and other factors that could affect their decision to relocate.

Only after this has been accomplished should the recruiter begin to "paint a picture" of the practice. During this portion of the screen, the recruiter must rely on the detailed practice and community assessments that have been completed prior to the search. It is at this point that the recruiter begins to "talk doctor," sharing the clinical and business aspects of the practice, revealing his understanding of the physician's specialty and his understanding of medical practice dynamics and economics.

This is the critical juncture where a recruiter earns his or her salt by gaining the physician's trust. It is intimate knowledge of the opportunity and the recruiter's ability to objectively present both the positives and potential negatives of the practice that will demonstrate to the physician that he is dealing with a professional. Knowledge of the practice, knowledge of the hospital, knowledge of the community – all these are critical when speaking to a class of professionals who put a premium on data and analysis.

The objective of the presentation at this point is to demonstrate to the physician that – despite any negatives – the opportunity can satisfy his or her professional and personal needs. If that is not the case, the recruiter should make this clear and suggest ways in which the physician could find an opportunity that is a better match. Such candor is far preferable to an attempt to "fit a round peg in a square hole." While putting a positive spin on a practice may lead to a physician interview, recruiters who try to force an inappropriate match are setting their organizations up for failure. The physician will see through this effort during the interview or, worse, shortly after he or she relocates to the practice.

Overcoming Objections

During the course of the conversation, physicians are likely to voice objections to the opportunity the recruiter is representing. For medical residents in particular, the objection almost inevitably has to do with geography. Younger physicians often have a very specific idea of where they wish to practice, and this usually is where they trained, where they grew up, where their spouse grew up, or where they would like to vacation. Their priorities rarely have to do with the dynamics of a practice, including specifics such as payer mix, path to partner, group governance, etc. That is why so many young physicians leave their initial practice setting within a year or two. Enamored with a particular location, they join practices that do not meet their needs or expectations and quickly become disillusioned. This phenomenon is not limited to young doctors. After all, how many people do you know who are still in their first jobs?

What the recruiter must do is pose this contradiction back to the candidate with a question similar to the following:

"Why, Dr. Jones, would you spend a dozen or more years in collegiate and post-collegiate training mastering the art of medicine, and then choose a practice based on its location rather than on the art you have sacrificed so much to learn?"

The candidate's first priority should be the practice. The recruiter must first help the candidate realize what is truly important to them in a medical setting. What type of earning potential do they need to meet their financial goals? What types of patients do they want to see? How much personal time do they need? What types of colleagues do they want to work with?

The practice is where they are going to spend the majority of their time and if their work environment does not suit them, they will not be satisfied.

Convincing residents of this fact is a challenge, because in general, they don't have a professional motivation for relocating – their motivation is largely a function of geographic preference. This is another reason why recruiters should not invest the majority of their time and energy pursuing residents.

In practice physicians, by contrast, often do have reasons to relocate that are professionally based. Having been in a medical practice, they understand the dynamics and have a clearer idea of the type of practice that suits them best. In such cases, the recruiter must understand the physician's motivation for seeking a new practice. In practice physicians also may have geographic preferences. However, by knowing the physician's motivations, recruiters can illustrate how the opportunity they represent matches those motivations, as in the following question:

"Dr. Jones, do you want to end up right back where you are, in a practice with high overhead, low reimbursement, and high malpractice rates? Our practice opportunity features low overhead, high reimbursement, and low malpractice…and the community has a lot of the same benefits provided by the location you prefer."

There are a variety of other objections that physicians will voice – perhaps the opportunity is not close to their family, or the climate is not ideal for them. Each of these objections often can be addressed if the practice and community offer most of what the physician needs.

Direct the Process

Once physicians are persuaded that an opportunity does offer the potential for a better quality of practice and life, they will begin to investigate the opportunity on their own. While this is occurring, the recruiter should stay in continual communication with the physician, sending them additional information about the practice and community and responding quickly to requests.

This is another stage in the process where time spent on the front end of the search can pay dividends. If the recruiting team has been set up properly and can communicate quickly, then the recruiter will be able to respond to physician requests in a timely manner. However, if the physician has questions about hospital procedures, standards of care, school policies or other matters, and the recruiter is unable to obtain timely, substantive, and accurate answers to these questions from the recruiting team, then credibility will be lost and distrust may develop.

With coordinated teamwork and access to information, the recruiter can help direct the process and not be voiceless as the physician seeks information independently and consults with his or her circle of advisers. In many cases, these advisers may not be working in the recruiter's best interest since likely as not they will want the physician to remain where they are. However, if the recruiter has prepared thoroughly and done his or her job well, he or she will have gained enough credibility that the candidate's initial interest in interviewing will be reaffirmed.

We are now one critical step closer to the tip of the iceberg – the point at which a physician has agreed to interview.

CHAPTER 15

THE INTERVIEW

An effective physician candidate interview is based on a clear understanding of what the interview is for. The interview should not be structured as an introduction to the opportunity. Rather, the candidate interview is a time for ***confirmation,*** not ***investigation.***

When the interview is properly arranged, both the recruiting party and the physician candidate are meeting to confirm information that each party has ***previously learned about the other.*** An effective physician candidate interview is based on hours of pre-interview conversations that have taken place with both the candidate and his or her spouse during the screening process.

The candidate will already know beforehand the basic terms of the offer. He or she will know what type of call schedule is in place, what the weekly work hours are, path to partnership, payer mix in the practice, and associated details. In turn, the recruiting party should have a written profile of the candidate, spouse and family in hand detailing their professional backgrounds and their personal interests. By preparing on the front end, the interview does not become a forum for protracted and possibly contentious ***negotiations***, but rather is an opportunity to ***connect on a personal basis.***

The "70/30" Rule.

For this reason, we believe the candidate interview should be structured to be ***70% social and 30% professional.***

The goal is to allow the candidate and his or her spouse to walk through the practice and the community and to visualize living and working there. ***It is imperative that the spouse be on the interview.*** If the spouse cannot make the interview, the interview should be rescheduled. Practice relocation is invariably a joint decision, and often the spouse is the ultimate decision maker. An interview without the spouse is usually wasted motion.

The candidate and spouse should be able to meet and socialize with people of their own age and interests to experience what life and practice is like in your community. Both the candidate and spouse should be provided with a written itinerary in advance that allows them to view the practice, the hospital, the schools, real estate and other places of interest.

At the same time, the recruiting party or parties need to observe the physician interacting with physicians, administrators, and other key stakeholders in the search in both professional and social settings. Stakeholders then can determine if the candidate is the kind of physician and the kind of person they can spend hours interacting with each day – and the kind of physician who will thrive in the community.

The interview itinerary should be customized to each physician, as follows:

Customized Interview Itinerary

- Candidate meets with doctors in the same specialty
- Candidate meets with referring physicians
- Candidate meets with newly recruited doctors
- Candidate meets with administrators/medical directors
- Candidate and spouse meet with people of similar age/interests
- Candidate and spouse meet with school representatives
- Candidate and spouse tour the community
- Candidate and spouse see/experience where they can enjoy their hobbies/recreational/cultural interests
- Separate itinerary for the spouse

Role of the Hospital CEO or Group Administrator

We have stated earlier that physician recruitment is a top strategic goal for hospitals and medical groups, and its importance to the success of medical organizations can hardly be overemphasized. For this reason, the hospital CEO or group administrator must be a champion of the recruiting process.

Direct participation by the CEO or administrator should begin before the interview when the CEO/Administrator establishes a sense of urgency and commitment in the physician recruiting team. The CEO/Administrator generally hands off the daily tactical duties to an in-house and/or an agency recruiter and other members of the recruiting team. However, he or she stays attuned to the process and leads by example, especially in the areas of accessibility and responsiveness.

This is particularly the case when it comes to scheduling physician interviews. Unfortunately, candidates are not always able to schedule interviews at times that are convenient to members of the recruiting team. Qualified candidates are at such a premium, however, that every effort should be made to meet their interview time-frames, even if some recruiting team members' personal activities need to be rearranged. The CEO/Administrator can set the tone by being accessible even when it may not be personally convenient.

During the interview, direct participation by the CEO/Administrator makes a positive impression on candidates and is usually essential to a positive result. Only the CEO/Administrator can break any logjams that may occur in terms of decision making, the dissemination of information, and other factors that can obstruct a search. The physician recruiter can only take the process so far. At some point, the leader of the organization has to put his or her stamp on the process.

What to Ask

While many details about the practice and the financial package should be reviewed in advance, there are issues you will want to confirm and discuss with the candidate during the interview. These questions will help eliminate ambiguity and help gauge the physicians' interest level and priorities. Sample questions include:

- What do you know about our practice?
- What more information do you need about our practice? (Confirm all relevant details re: finances, call, hours, etc.)
- What interests you about our opportunity?
- What are your expectations for our practice?
- What do you need to provide optimum care to your patients?
- What would a good day be like in your ideal practice?
- What is the culture like in your current practice?
- Are there any specialty areas you would like to focus on?
- What assets do you think you would bring to our group?
- What would you like or expect from the hospital?
- What are your goals for the next 3-5 years?
- What do you know about our community?
- What other information would you like about our community?
- Is there any further information we can provide to your spouse?
- Have you scheduled other interviews?
- What interests you about the other opportunities you are considering?

- What is your time frame for making a decision?
- Are your initial expectations for the opportunity consistent with what you have actually seen and heard during this interview?
- Now that the interview is over, do you still have a strong interest in our opportunity?

These and related questions are meant to ensure that the candidate is fully informed about the opportunity. They also will help determine if the candidate's expectations are consistent with what the opportunity actually offers.

Role of the Realtor

Real estate is a critical factor for anyone considering a move. Candidate interviews generally include a tour of community real estate options guided by a local realtor. Hospitals and medical groups should choose carefully among local realtors to find an exemplary professional to work with. The realtor should understand that their role in the interview is not truly about real estate. ***Their primary role is to act as a community advocate.*** The realtor should understand that the physician and his or her spouse have not yet made a decision to join the community. They will be seeking information from the realtor as a third party not directly affiliated with the recruiting hospital or group. The realtor is so important to the process that Merritt, Hawkins & Associates' recruiting consultants often accompany realtors on a "trial tour" of the community prior to the interview to ensure that they understand their role and are able to present the community in a positive light.

Be wary of realtors whose goal is to sell the most expensive house in their portfolios. Make sure they understand the type of house and financial parameters of the candidate and spouse and that they stay within those parameters. We have had many occasions where physicians visiting smaller communities with excellent real estate values have told us after the interview that they liked the community but could not afford to buy a house there. Unfortunately, the realtor had only shown them the two or three most expensive houses in town.

In selecting a realtor, consider that candidates typically will spend one hour interviewing with a peer physician but two to three hours touring the community with a realtor. The realtor therefore is a critical representative of the community who must be aligned with the other members of the recruiting team. Realtors also can provide excellent feedback regarding the candidate's interest in the community.

References

The extent and depth of references needed to schedule a candidate interview are not as great as those needed to credential a physician at the local hospital or hospitals. Some hospitals and groups make the mistake of insisting on a complete referencing and credentialing process prior to scheduling the interview. The problem with this strategy is that candidates usually are fielding multiple offers. The long delays that can take place in the referencing process can cost a hospital or group the chance to interview the candidate in their opportunity. In addition, at this stage of the process some candidates may not have told colleagues or patients that they may be leaving the practice and as a result may be reluctant to furnish local references until they are certain that a deal will be consummated.

In some cases, candidates who interview may later be dropped from consideration based on what happens during the referencing and credentialing process. That is an unfortunate waste of time and money. However, hospitals and groups that invest an inordinate amount of time investigating candidates before they interview can undermine their ability to recruit effectively, which in the long run is an even greater waste of time and money.

One Interview Only

Through extensive front-end preparation, and by involving the spouse the first time, only one candidate interview should be necessary. Typically, the interview will take place over a 24 – 48 hour period. Limiting candidate interviews saves money but it also motivates all parties to make a maximum effort. Nothing can be left to chance when everyone concerned knows they have one time to get it right. In our experience, everyone puts their best foot forward when it is understood that the process is limited to one interview.

It is during the interview that the recruiting hospital or group has an opportunity to distinguish itself based on a superior level of commitment. Whether it's in sports, business, or medicine, those recruiters who show that they "want it more" generally win out. Physicians have told us on countless occasions that they selected a particular practice based mostly on the attitude of the people recruiting them. That's why it never hurts to "pull out all the stops." Signs welcoming the physician and spouse in the lobby of the hospital, a small gift in the hotel room, a short visit with the swimming coach or piano instructor -- if one of the physician's children is interested in these activities – all of this extra effort will leave the physician and spouse with that warm feeling of being wanted that is so critical to successful recruitment.

If the candidate appears to be a positive match, it is important to state at the end of the interview that they did well, that you are favorably impressed with them, and that you are greatly interested in having them join the practice and the community. It also is appropriate to ask the physician about his or her level of interest. As stated above, the question may be phrased: "Now that you have seen our practice and community, do you still have a strong interest in joining us?"

The way the candidate responds to this question often will tell you more than what he or she actually says. It also is appropriate to stress to the candidate the importance of physician recruitment to the hospital or group and that the process cannot be put on hold while the candidate is making a decision. This is not to pressure the candidate. It is simply to make clear that a timely decision is required, whether or not that decision is yes or no.

Once the interview is over, all the recruiting party can do is wait for the candidate to make his or her decision. Right?

Wrong. We have now come to the moment of truth in the physician recruiting process – what we call "The Pyramid of Interest" -- which is the topic of the next chapter.

CHAPTER 16

THE PYRAMID OF INTEREST

In the previous chapter, we discussed how there is a distinct psychological progression from the point at which a recruiter first contacts a candidate to the point at which the candidate has gained enough trust in the recruiter to schedule an interview.

There also is a distinct psychological progression from the point at which the interview concludes to the point at which the candidate either accepts the offer and signs a contract, or declines the offer and moves on. We call this progression the "Pyramid of Interest." The diagrams below illustrate the concept.

Interest Builds

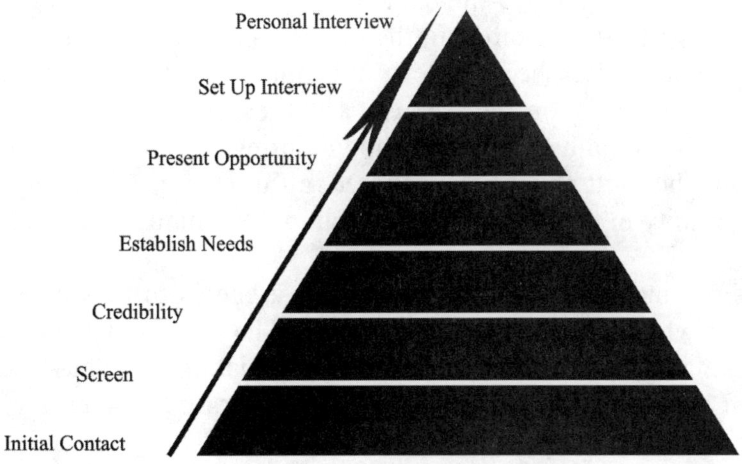

Interest Peaks

Interest Declines

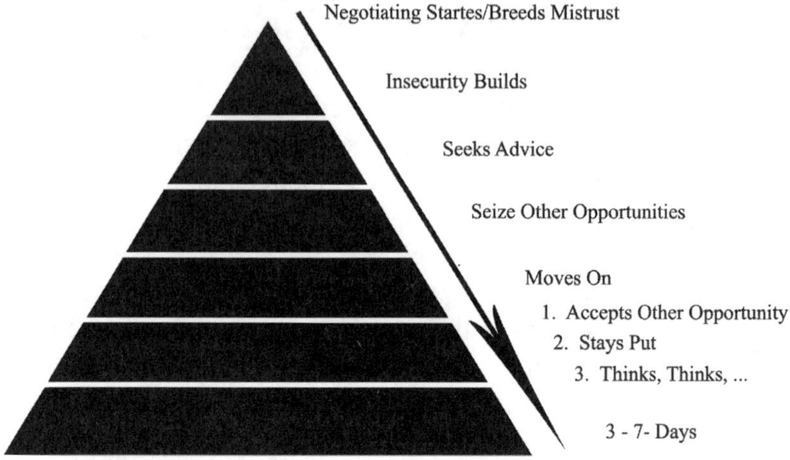

The first diagram shows the meticulous process of trust-building necessary to schedule and conduct the on-site candidate interview. Diagram two illustrates that the candidate's interest in the opportunity peaks during the 48 hour period immediately after the interview. It is during this two-day window that the candidate and his or her spouse are the most enthused about relocating. All the hospitality they were shown during the interview, all the positive vibrations they felt about being wanted, all the things that interested them in the opportunity in the first place are fresh in their minds.

The third diagram indicates how this peak interest begins to fade and may dilute to the point where the candidate moves on. The trigger that starts the downward slide almost always has to do with negotiation. Because some contractual point was not addressed either before or during the interview, or because there was poor communication among the recruiting team on the front end of the recruiting process, a negotiation of some kind develops after the candidate has interviewed and returned home.

There are a variety of negotiation points that may arise. Perhaps the recruiting team never clearly laid out the terms of potential buy-in to the practice. It is only *after* the interview that they inform the physician candidate that part of the buy-in includes a "blue sky" provision. Similarly, other aspects of the practice, such as work hours, call schedules or vacation times might not have been finalized by the recruiting team in time for the interview. When these important details are communicated to the candidate after the interview, he or she may feel misled.

Once negotiating starts, distrust can begin to build on both sides. The candidate then will seek advice. Friends and peers will weigh in with cautionary tales about doctors who have gotten into bad deals, or they may start to erode the candidate's enthusiasm about the geographic area in which the opportunity is located.

While this is taking place, the rest of the world is not standing still. It is likely that the candidate is receiving solicitations from other recruiters who are trying to persuade them to "just look at one more opportunity" before they get back to the people with whom they recently interviewed. We know this because, frankly, it often is our recruiters who are calling doctors who have recently interviewed at locations we do not represent and are in the negotiating process.

The end result is that the candidate takes another opportunity, decides to stay put, or simply delays making a decision indefinitely and the recruiting party is obliged to break off negotiations and move on.

In our experience, within the single interview framework, if the candidate does not commit to the opportunity ***within three to seven days***, it is unlikely that he or she ever will. It therefore is imperative to bring the recruitment to a close during this crucial one week period. But how?

The Three C's – Contract, Communication, Commitment

In a Broadway production, the play is over when the curtain goes down. Given all the effort that goes into making it happen, a physician interview can feel like a Broadway show. Once the interview is over, the "cast" may heave a collective sigh of relief and there is a tendency to let down. Unfortunately, the urgency that went into making the interview happen often does not continue into the "closing" process.

The physician contract is a critical component of the closing process, and this is one area where the ball often is dropped. As we alluded to earlier, ***a sample contract must be in place prior to the interview,*** even if some changes to the contract must be made post-interview. There is no other way for the physician to make a binding commitment other than to sign a contract. After the interview, the final, executable contract should be provided to the physician immediately.

Indeed, our recruiters make a point of personally flying to the candidate's community, when possible, with a copy of the final contract to sign. This "signing trip" ensures a speedy commitment and reinforces to the physician the sense of urgency the recruiting hospital or medical group feels about his or her decision to relocate. It prepares the physician for what is going to come next, including hearing from patients who may be upset that he or she is going to leave and hearing from physician partners who may try to enhance the doctor's status in the group so that he or she will not leave. A counter-proposal is a compliment, but the physician should be reminded that his or her reasons for leaving may not all be financial. Physicians also should be reminded that they had to "quit" before being offered a more desirable situation.

Given what is often at stake in physician recruitment, we do not feel that it is superfluous to personally send recruiters to the physician's home to make sure that the lengthy, labor intensive process of recruitment comes to a positive close.

Communication is another key component in the closing process. It is easy to pay lip service to the importance of communication, but in practice many hospitals and medical groups are not as zealous about following up with candidates as they should be. Communication ***does not mean a hard sell.*** It is counterproductive to try to badger physicians into making a decision. However, as we referenced earlier, it is appropriate to make clear to candidates during the interview that the hospital or medical group would appreciate a timely decision.

Follow-up communication should be geared toward providing candidates with any additional information they need to make an informed decision. If the Recruiting Committee has been set up properly, it will be able to relay additional information about the practice, schools, real estate and other matters back to the candidate within days if not hours.

In order to maintain the good feelings of the first 48 hours post-interview, candidates should be contacted on a near daily basis, either by phone, email or text message. There are several ways in which positive momentum can be maintained, including:

- ♦ Have a physician call the candidate and express how eager he or she is to have the candidate join the practice.

- ♦ Have a member of the Recruiting Committee call the spouse directly to discuss school, recreational or other areas about which the spouse has expressed interest.

- ♦ Have the hospital CEO or group administrator call the candidate and reiterate how much he or she is needed in the community. Remember, "little things" count. Flowers or a gift basket with locally produced items accompanied by a personal note can go a long way toward tipping the balance in your favor.

The third "C" – commitment – must be present throughout the recruiting process. Commitment means devoting the energy, resources and time necessary to see the recruitment through to a positive conclusion. Post-interview, commitment may mean being available to speak to candidates after hours, or coming to the table with the extra incentive that may be the only thing delaying a doctor from signing a contract. Commitment is an intangible, but often is the most critical component in a successful physician search.

A Process, Not an Event

Congratulations. After a considerable amount of effort structuring the search, screening candidates, and conducting interviews, the candidate has signed a contract and has committed to joining you. Still, the recruiting process is not over. There are licensing and credentialing issues to consider, in addition to ensuring the physician is signed up with various insurance plans and networks. The hospital and/or group must stay in continual communication with the candidate through this process, helping to obtain necessary information so that the physician does not become discouraged or second guess his or her decision.

When the physician does relocate, he or she must be assimilated into the community through practice marketing, which usually will include. Then the process of retention begins, in conjunction with the beginning of the next physician search that is required.

The point is that physician recruitment is a continuous cycle, not an isolated event with a discrete beginning, middle and end. Hospitals and medical groups that succeed in maintaining and enhancing their medical staffs are in constant recruitment mode, both planning for the long-term and capable of responding quickly to any immediate recruiting challenges.

Our discussion of how to recruit physicians ends here. In the following chapters we review two subjects that will play an ever more important role in the physician recruiting process.

The first is temporary, or *locum tenens,* physician staffing. The second is U.S. immigration laws and regulations.

CHAPTER 17

THE ROLE OF LOCUM TENENS

Most people are not used to thinking of physicians as "temps." Nevertheless, a significant number of doctors in the United States today work on a temporary, or *locum tenens,* basis. This is an important trend to consider as temporary physician staffing and permanent physician recruitment become more interconnected.

The use of temporary, *locum tenens* physicians dates from the mid-1970's. Locum tenens (the term, roughly translated from Latin, means "holding a place") initially were used by hospitals and medical groups primarily to provide coverage for doctors on vacation or those pursuing continuing medical education (CME).

At first, physicians working on a locum tenens basis were not always judged favorably by their peers or by health care administrators. The perception (and sometimes the reality) was that locum tenens physicians were compromised in some way and so could not maintain permanent, full-time practices. There were only a handful of physicians working on a locum tenens basis at that time.

Locum tenens took a great leap forward in the mid 1990s, when the advent of managed care put a premium on primary care "gatekeeper" physicians. There was a virtual feeding frenzy in the industry in which hospitals and medical groups were feverishly attempting to create networks of physician gatekeepers who would control patient entry into the health care system. If permanent physicians could not be found immediately, many medical groups and hospitals turned to locum tenens doctors to "hold a place" until permanent physicians could be recruited.

The gatekeeper system ultimately fizzled in most parts of the country (taking many physician practice management firms with it), and demand for primary care physicians significantly abated. However, another trend developed which has kept demand for locum tenens rising. Enhanced medical technology, population growth and population aging created a shortage of specialist physicians that began in the mid 1990s and has accelerated ever since. The shortage has driven the use of locum tenens doctors continuously upward.

The following numbers are derived from an annual survey of the locum tenens market conducted by Staff Care, a firm specializing in locum tenens staffing (like Merritt, Hawkins & Associates, Staff Care is a division of AMN Healthcare.) **Note: Staff Care's 2006 Review is included in this book.** Several numbers from the survey reflect the rising use of locum tenens.

Estimated Annual Spending on Temporary Physician Staffing

2005	2004	2003	2002	2001
$3.2 billion	$2.9 billion	$2.6 billion	$1.93 billion	$1.25 billion

Source: Staff Care, 2006 Review of Temporary Physician Staffing Trends

The growth of locum tenens also can be measured by the number of physicians working on a locum tenens basis, (see below):

Estimated Number of Physicians Working Locum Tenens

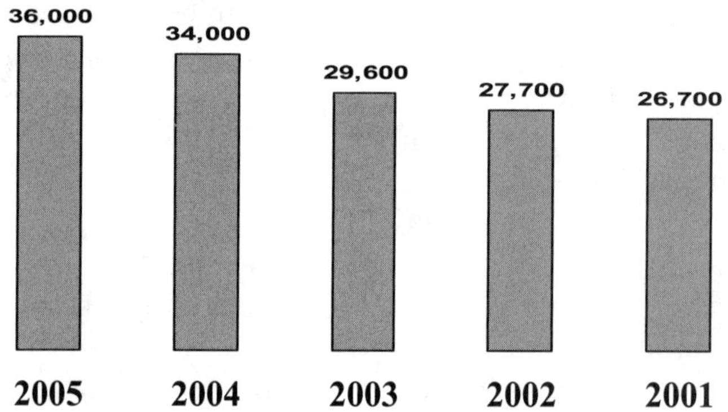

Source: Staff Care, Inc. 2006 Review of Temporary Physician Staffing Trends

The increasing use of locum tenens suggests a growing acceptance of locum tenens physicians among physicians, health care administrators, and patients. Part of this acceptance is a function of the malpractice crisis, which has greatly increased the level of scrutiny to which locum tenens physicians are subjected. The privileging process for locum tenens physicians has become very rigorous, in many cases as rigorous as privileging newly recruited permanent physicians. The Review of Temporary Physician Staffing Trends referenced above includes interviews with hospital and medical group administrators who were asked about the current acceptance of locum tenens doctors (see the following):

How are Locum Tenens Providers Viewed at Your Facility By:

	Accepted	Not Accepted	Tolerated	Unsure
Permanent medical providers	74%	0%	16%	10%
Administrators	77%	1%	15%	7%
Patients	65%	1%	17%	17%

Source: Staff Care 2006 Review of Temporary Physician Staffing Trends

Acceptance of locum tenens physicians also is rising because new categories of physicians are being attracted to locum tenens practices. Successful older physicians find locum tenens to be appealing because much of the third party payer "hassle factors" that they object to are eliminated. For younger physicians, locum tenens provides a convenient way to experiment with various practice settings before choosing a permanent practice.

In many medical specialties, the number of permanent recruitment candidates is decreasing due to a variety of factors, including physician retirement, the preference among younger doctors for a controllable lifestyle, and immigration policies that are limiting the number of international medical graduates. The number of locum tenens candidates, by contrast, is growing, prompting health care executives to find new uses for this increasingly important source of physicians.

Multiple Uses For Locum Tenens

As hospitals and medical group managers review their strategies for recruiting permanent physician candidates, it is important to also consider how locum tenens physicians can be used as part of a comprehensive medical staff plan.

There are a variety of ways in which locum tenens can play a complementary role in physician staff planning. These include:

- *Vacation and CME coverage.* This traditional use of locum tenens has not diminished in recent years and has, in fact, increased, due to reasons referenced earlier. Many younger physicians are seeking practices that offer set vacations, regular hours, and favorable coverage schedules. In addition, the number of female physicians has increased dramatically in recent years, and many female physicians require time off because of their dual roles as professionals and homemakers. The number of locum tenens "physician days" needed to cover vacation time is running into the millions per year.

Some hospitals and medical groups are inclined to simply work their physicians harder or influence their doctors away from taking their allotted vacation time. Others use locum tenens providers to ensure that physicians are able to take vacations as promised. This serves as both a recruiting tool, helping some hospitals and groups achieve a reputation for being "physician-friendly" and as a retention tool during a time when physician turnover is particularly hard to address.

- *Place-holder while a permanent search is ongoing.* The physician shortage has left many hospitals, medical groups and other facilities under-staffed. A growing number of facilities are using locum tenens doctors to maintain services and revenue until permanent candidates can be recruited. In its 2006 Review, Staff Care asked hospital and medical group administrators why they use locum tenens physicians. More administrators cited "to hold a place until permanent staff is recruited" than any other factor.

- *Physician retirement or disability.* About one third of physicians in the U.S. today are 55 or older, and abrupt physician retirements are not uncommon. When an established physician suddenly turns in his or her stethoscope, locum tenens physicians can maintain continuity of care until the practice can reorganize and adjust. The same is true in cases of physician disability.

- *Test marketing new service lines.* Many hospitals wish to experiment with new services but hesitate to recruit new physicians full-time in case a viable market does not exist. Some hospitals use locum tenens physicians to gauge patient receptiveness to new services and can then make a more informed decision regarding whether or not to add the service.

- *Expanding into new market areas.* Hospitals seeking to establish satellite clinics may not wish to gamble by recruiting a permanent physician to set up practice in a new location. Instead, they staff the clinic with one or more locum tenens physicians to establish a foothold in the area. If the practice proves viable, they then can recruit a permanent doctor.

- *Enhance permanent physician recruiting efforts.* Hospitals and medical groups can use locum tenens physicians to bolster their permanent physician recruiting efforts. A locums physician can build a patient base so that when a permanent physician joins the community he or she can hit the ground running. In addition, a locums physician with a thriving patient load demonstrates clearly to permanent recruitment candidates that a sound practice really exists. In addition, it is not unusual for locum tenens physicians to see the advantages of working for a particular hospital or group and to join the staff full-time.

- *Prevent patient defections.* Health care today is becoming more consumer driven, and "customer service" has become a greater priority. During flu season or peak usage periods locum tenens physicians can handle patient overflow and forestall patients who might grow impatient from lengthy appointments and seek care elsewhere.

- *Secure larger managed care accounts.* Hospitals and medical groups seeking large managed care accounts often are reluctant or unable to recruit a significant number of permanent physicians until the account has been secured. However, they cannot secure such accounts until they can demonstrate they have the staff to service the account. By working with a pool of locum tenens physicians, they can demonstrate to the account that they have the necessary manpower and be sure of the account before they recruit permanent physicians.

- *Hospital expansion.* As hospitals expand, they often allow groups to bid on hospital based services such as radiology or anesthesiology. Groups that may not have the current manpower to handle the hospital's increased volumes can supplement their staffs with locum tenens physicians and remain competitive in the bidding process.

- *Maintain revenue.* Hospitals and groups considering locum tenens must take a close look at the potential return on investment. While locum tenens physicians are a cost, this cost must be weighed against the revenue locum tenens physicians generate. In some cases, locum tenens physicians more than pay for themselves by maintaining revenues for the hospital or group.

- *Continuity of care.* Last, but not least, quality of care is largely dependent on continuity. Locum tenens physicians can maintain continuity of care for patients when current levels of physician manpower are insufficient.

Hospitals and medical groups that consistently use locum tenens physicians often develop a “pool” of practitioners who are familiar with the group’s geographic area and their style of practice. This pool acts a “reserve unit” capable of filling in on short notice in a variety of scenarios.

By using locum tenens physicians strategically, hospitals and medical groups are better positioned to respond to a market where permanent physicians are in increasingly short supply.

CHAPTER 18

IMMIGRATION FAQ

As we referenced earlier, one-quarter of physicians in active patient care in the United States today are international medical graduates (IMGs). Many of these physicians came to the United States to train on one of several types of visas. Hospitals, medical groups, and other employers must deal with U.S. immigration laws in order to recruit from this pool of candidates. Some understanding of these laws often proves useful for physician recruiters.

Following are a number of frequently asked questions concerning U.S. immigration laws as they pertain to international medical graduates. The questions and answers were prepared by Carl Shusterman, a prominent immigration attorney based in Los Angeles. Mr. Shusterman's web site (www.shusterman.com) contains a wealth of information about immigration law and is a useful resource for physician, nurse and other recruiters.

What Is An International Medical Graduate (IMG?)

Any person, U.S. citizen or otherwise, who attended a non-U.S. or a non-Canadian medical school.

How Many IMGs Are There?

Close to 200,000. Roughly one-quarter of physicians in active patient care are IMGs. In some specialties, such as the following, they represent more than one-quarter of active physicians.

Anesthesiology	31%
Cardiology	30%
IM	32%
Nephrology	40%
Psychiatry	31%

How Many Residents Are IMGs?

Over 23,000 residents come out of U.S. residency training each year. About 5,000 are IMGs.

Why Consider Them?

Apart from the numbers, IMGs have gained greater acceptance among administrators, patients and doctors. Many department heads, medical directors, heads of medical societies and top specialists are IMGs. By considering IMGs, hospitals, medical groups and other entities seeking physicians can expand the candidate pool without sacrificing quality.

What Must IMGs Do To Practice In The U.S.?

A system is in place to ensure that IMGs have the same skill sets as U.S. or Canadian graduates. To practice in the U.S., IMGs must:

- Obtain the Educational Council of Foreign Medical Graduates (ECFMG) Certificate showing equivalent knowledge to U.S./Canadian med school graduates.

- To get an ECFMG Certificate they must pass USMLE I and II, and pass the ECFMG English language test. USMLE Part II has been split into two parts: CK (Clinical Knowledge) and CS (Clinical Skills) so that the old Clinical Skills Assessment (CSA) test is no longer given.

- They can take USMLE Part III after one year of residency. Those wanting to enter the U.S. to do a residency on H-1B status must have taken and passed USMLE I, II and III and received their ECFMG certification.

- Must complete a U.S. based residency program.

Not all IMGs who apply for ECFMG Certification can pass the tests. Generally, only the best physicians from other countries are able to meet the necessary qualifications.

What Is A J-1 Visa?

It is a visa for those seeking education/training in the U.S. and is sponsored by the Education Commission for Foreign Medical Graduates (ECFMG). It gives the holder up to 7 years to complete graduate medical education (GME)

However, once GME is completed, the holder ***must return to his or her country for 2 years or obtain a waiver of the two-year home residency requirement through an Interested Government Agency.***

What Is A J Waiver?

A J waiver gets the J-1 visa holder out of the two-year post-residency requirement to return to his or her country.

To get a waiver, the J doctor must be sponsored by an "Interested Government Agency" and obtain a job in a federally designated Health Professional Shortage Area (HPSA) or a Medically Underserved Area (MUA).

Effective fiscal year 2005, some states are issuing up to 5 waivers to physicians who are not working in underserved areas, but serve a large underserved population. The policy is mainly to help medical centers in large urban areas that are not in an underserved area but serve a large number of indigents. Examples of this are some teaching hospitals in New York City.

In a very limited number of cases, an IMG also can obtain a J waiver if leaving the country would cause the doctor's United States Citizen or Permanent Resident spouse or children to suffer exceptional hardship. Exceptional hardship waivers are extremely difficult to obtain, unless the physician's U.S. citizen child or spouse has an illness that cannot be treated in the home country or the political situation in the home country is dangerous to the well being of the child and/or spouse.

How Can I Find Out If My Facility Is In A HPSA Or MUA?

Contact Ellie Najfabadi at Carl Shusterman's office at 213-623-4592. Provide her with the facility location (complete address of the location/s where the physician will be employed, including zip code).

Both urban and rural areas can be HPSAs/MUAs. An individual hospital can be an MUA, but the physician has to actually work in an office located in an HPSA/MUA.

What Government Agencies Sponsor J Waivers?

- The Veterans Administration……VA facilities - primary care and specialists
- The Delta Regional Authority….primary care and specialists, Mississippi Delta states only see – www.dra.gov
- Department of Health and Human Services…Primary care only, very few hospitals qualify (the location where the physician will be employed must have a HPSA designation score of 7 or higher.) In addition, the employer must be a FQHC clinic. Few employers qualify. Limited to community health centers located in qualified areas.
- The Appalachian Regional Commission……Primary care doctors and psychiatrists only, only in the Appalachian states

What Is The "Conrad 30" Program?

Not only federal agencies can sponsor doctors for J waivers. Each state Department of Health can participate in the Conrad 30 program, sponsored by Kent Conrad, a senator from North Dakota, and Senator Sam Brownback of Kansas. The program allows each state to sponsor 30 J doctors for waivers each year.

As of now, all 50 states are participating.

All participating states have slots for primary care and specialists, except California, which only has slots for primary care.

What Happens If The State Has Used Up Its Quota Of 30 J Waivers?

States vary as to when the quota period begins and some states do use up their annual numbers quickly – so this is an important factor to check. If the numbers are used up, no more will be available until the next quota period begins.

What Happens Once A J Physician Gets A Waiver?

The physician "adjusts his status" to an H-1B temporary work visa and must work for a particular employer in a HPSA or MUA for 3 years.

Can The J Physician, Now On An H-1B, Change Employers?

Only if the employer terminates the H-1B doctor or violates the terms of the doctor's contract and only if the new employer is in a HPSA/MUA.

Does The Doctor Have To Be An Employee And Does An Income Guarantee Show Employee/Employer Status?

The physician has to be sponsored as an employee. This can be the group, hospital, an individual doctor, or some other entity acting as the physician's employer. However, for immigration purposes, the group can be the employer even if the hospital is fronting the income guarantee.

Can IMGs Start Residency On Any Other Kind Of Visa Besides The J-1?

Yes. Some IMGs can enter U.S. residency on H-1B visas, the temporary visa for foreign professionals. They must pass the same requirements as J physicians, only they must have passed USMLE Part III before applying for H-1B status with the Center for Immigration Services (CIS.). The H-1B is good for the duration of the program, not to exceed six years, though under narrow exceptions, a physician can extend his H-1B status longer than six years.

The H-1B is an "employer-sponsored" visa, so to get one a foreign professional must find a U.S. employer to sponsor them.

In the case of doctors, the sponsor is the residency program.

Can Medical Facilities Use IMGs Who Are Completing Their Residency On H-1Bs?

Yes – all the physician needs is an offer of employment, and they can "transfer" from one employer (the residency program) to another (the medical facility.). ***The employer does not have to be in a HPSA or MUA.***

However, the doctor ***must be able to obtain a green card before the H-1B expires.*** If the doctor gets out of residency with 2 or 3 years left on his H-1B, in most cases he will be able to obtain a green card before his H-1B expires. Even if the H-1B expires, an extension is possible. In most cases, Mr. Shusterman's office can find a way to get a doctor who trained on an H-

1B a green card, even if they do not have a great deal of time left on their H-1B.

How Long Does It Take For An H-1B Doctor Completing Residency To "Transfer" His H-1B From One Employer To Another?

To get an H-1B, the doctor must have passed USMLE I, II & III and be licensed in the state where he'll be working. Once licensure is obtained, it then takes about 30-90 days for the H-1B to come through, ***unless*** the doctor or the employer wants to pay for "Premium Processing", in which case the H-1B is guaranteed in 15 days. "Premium Processing" costs $1,000.

Isn't There An Annual H-1B Quota?

Yes. The government will issue 65,000 H-1Bs per year. This is an important point because this 65,000 cap is often reached very quickly – ***except for J waiver doctors, who are not subject to the cap, and for physicians working for academic institutions.***

What Does It Take To Get A Green Card?

Whether the doctor was on a J-1, but now is working in H-1B status, or whether they transferred their H-1B from their residency and now are working in H-1B status, they will need to get a green card.

There are several ways to do this – the standard way is by going through PERM – a process of proving that no U.S. citizen or permanent resident is qualified, willing or able to take the job. This requires advertising in a major daily paper in the community where the doctor will be working and advertising in a major medical journal for the job (usually in JAMA). This process takes considerably less time than it used to.

More time can be removed from the process through the "National Interest Waiver" though this ***only works for doctors (Primary Care and Specialists) working in underserved areas.*** It is not necessary to run ads for the job to obtain a National Interest Waiver. To get a National Interest Waiver it's important to show that the employer is in ***a HPSA or a MUA and the employer is willing to give the physician a five-year contract. The physician can also open his or her own practice in an underserved area and receive an income guarantee from the hospital.***

Is There A Quota On Green Cards?

Yes, but most countries don't use their quota so backlogs are not a concern in many cases.

What Is An "O" Visa?

This is a visa for foreign superstars in their profession. For a doctor to get one they have to have a stellar publishing record – the bar is very high.

What About Canadian Physicians?

Canadian doctors are a different ballgame. They are not IMGs. The Canadian exam (LMCC) is reciprocated for licensure in some 40+ U.S. states.

However, to get an H-1B, **Canadian doctors must have a U.S. qualifying exam – the USMLE, FLEX, or the NBME.**

If they do, and once they obtain licensure in the relevant state, they can be in and working in as little as two weeks, **(but only if the annual H-1B quota has not been used up)** and the employer or physician is willing to pay a $1,000 fee for "Premium Processing."

Once they are on the H-1B they then can apply for a green card.

Can Canadians Practice In The U.S. Without A U.S. Exam?

Yes. Interestingly, U.S. employers can sponsor Canadian doctors for a green card, even if they have no U.S. exam. In other words, Canadians must have a U.S. exam to get a temporary, H-1B visa, but do not need a U.S. exam to get a green card, which allows them to stay here for life.

In the past, the problem has been that if a U.S. employer sponsors a Canadian doctor for a green card without going through the H-1B first, the time frame to get a green card was quite long – years, in some cases. ***But this has changed.***

It now takes about 12-18 months from the date the labor application is filed for a Canadian doctor with ***no U.S. exam*** to get a green card. This is quite workable in some cases, so the time is right for health facilities to consider the Canadian market.

Keep in mind that a growing number of young Canadian doctors are taking the USMLE because they know they need it to get an H-1B, another reason the Canadian market has become more favorable.

What Should You Do To Avoid Immigration Problems?

You don't want to get very far down the road with an IMG or a Canadian physician without having their case reviewed by an experienced immigration attorney. ***Make sure the doctor has a clear path to immigration!***

Each case is different with multiple immigration strategies available. In some cases, the doctor will have a problem that makes them an unviable candidate. Others may not seem like they are viable, but a competent attorney may be able to find a way.

For a comprehensive video discussion of physician immigration issues see Mr. Shusterman's online video presentation at:

http://shusterman.com/video/kaplan-img.ram.

SURVEYS

Following are the result of three surveys conducted by Merritt, Hawkins & Associates and Staff Care

Merritt, Hawkins & Associates®
2007 Review of Physician Recruitment Incentives

Merritt, Hawkins & Associates®
2007 Physician Inpatient/Outpatient Revenue Survey

Staff Care®
2006 Review of Temporary Physician Staffing Trends

Merritt Hawkins & Associates®

SUMMARY REPORT
2007 REVIEW OF PHYSICIAN AND CRNA RECRUITING INCENTIVES

OVERVIEW

Merritt Hawkins & Associates is a national health care search and consulting firm specializing in the recruitment of physicians in all medical specialties, as well as select allied health professionals. Established in 1987, Merritt Hawkins & Associates is a division of AMN Healthcare (NYSE: AHS) the nation's largest health care staffing organization and a Joint Commission-certified corporation. AMN Healthcare is comprised of 13 distinct health care staffing divisions and employs over 2,000 corporate employees in 12 domestic and seven international offices.

This report marks Merritt Hawkins & Associates 14th annual review of the search and consulting assignments we conduct on behalf of our clients.

The 2007 review is based on 3,016 physician, certified registered nurse anesthetist (CRNA) and select allied professional search and consulting assignments conducted by Merritt Hawkins & Associates from April 1, 2006 to March 31, 2007.

The intent of the review is to quantify financial and other incentives offered by our clients to physician and CRNA candidates during recruitment. The range of incentives detailed in the review may be used as one benchmark for evaluating which recruitment incentives are customary and competitive in today's physician and CRNA job market. The review is based on a national sample of search assignments and provides an indication of which medical specialties are currently in the greatest demand.

All of the following numbers are rounded to the nearest full digit.

Total Number of Physician and CRNA Search Assignments Represented:

2006/07	2005/06	2004/05	2003/04
3,016	2,840	2,687	2,594

Medical Settings of Physician Search Assignments

	2006/07	2005/06	2004/05	2003/04
Hospital	1,297 (43%)	654 (23%)	510 (19%)	285 (11%)
Group	1,058 (35%)	1,136 (40%)	1,290 (48%)	1,089 (42%)
Solo	244 (8 %)	483 (17%)	492 (18%)	519 (20%)
Partnership	238 (8%)	454 (16%)	242 (9%)	571 (22%)
Association	99 (3%)	28 (1%)	48 (2%)	78 (3%)
Other	74 (2%)	85 (3%)	105 (4%)	52 (2%)
HMO	6 (1%)	0 (0%)	0 (0%)	0 (0%)

Forty-eight States Where Search Assignments Were Conducted

AK, AL, AR, AZ, CA, CO, CT, FL, GA, IA, ID, IL, IN, KS, KY, LA, MA, MD, ME, MI, MO, MN, MS, MT, NC, ND, NE, NH, NJ, NM, NY, NV, OH, OK, OR, PA, RI,SC, SD, TN, TX, UT, VA, VT, WA, WI, WV, WY

Number of Searches by Community Size

	2006/07	2005/06	2004/05	2003/04
0-25,000	935 (31%)	769 (27%)	806 (30%)	622 (24%)
25,001-100,000	878 (29%)	935 (33%)	860 (32%)	960 (37%)
100,001+	1,203 (40%)	1,136 (40%)	1,021 (38%)	1,012 (39%)

Top 20 Physician Searches by Medical Specialty and CRNA Searches

	2006/07	2005/06	2004/05	2003/04
Family Practice*	303	257	166	165
Internal Medicine	273	274	188	124
Hospitalist	194	112	62	82
Radiology	187	237	218	202
Orthopedic Surgery	172	207	210	210
Cardiology	163	174	231	181
OB/GYN	159	111	83	103
General Surgery	121	165	116	112
Emergency Medicine	91	91	47	42
Psychiatry	81	69	80	54
Gastroenterology	78	105	94	105
Urology	63	75	59	94
Pediatrics	63	41	48	52
CRNA	61	117	102	82
HEM/ONC	59	45	n/a	n/a
Neurology	58	69	56	60
Otolaryngology	56	57	54	52
Anesthesiology	46	70	64	98
Dermatology	45	39	N/A	N/A
NeuroSurgery	41	50	61	52

*Includes Family Practice/Obstetrics

Top Five Specialties by Growth in Number of Search Assignments from 2005/06 - 2006/07

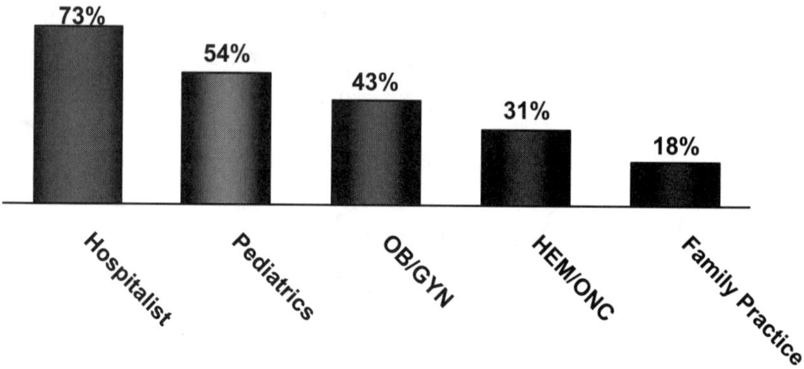

Other Specialty Recruitment Assignments

(Physician only, does not include allied professionals)

Allergy
Bariatric Surgery
Cardio-Electro Physiology
Cardiothoracic Surgery
Cardiovascular Surgery
Child Psychiatry
Critical Care/Pediatrics
Critical Care/Pulmonology
Endocrinology
Endovascular Surgery
Geriatrics
Gynecology
Gynecology/Oncology
Hand Surgery
Infectious Disease
Internal Medicine/Pediatrics
Maternal/Fetal Medicine
Musculo-Skeletal Radiology
Neonatology
Nephrology
Neurointensivist
Neurophysiology
Occupational Medicine
Ophthalmology
Oral Maxillofacial Surgery
Orthopedic Foot & Ankle Surgery
Orthopedic Hand Surgery
Orthopedic Spine Surgery
Orthopedic Total Joint
Orthopedic Trauma Surgery
Pain Management
Pathology
Pediatric Emergency Medicine
Pediatric HEM/ONC
Pediatric Neurologist
Pediatric Urology
Pediatric/Anesthesiology
Pediatric/Cardiology
Pediatric/Endocrinology
Pediatric/Intensivist
Pediatric/Nephrology
Pediatric/Radiology
Pediatric/Surgery
Perinatology
Physiatry
Plastic Surgery
Radiation Oncology
Rheumatology
Sleep Medicine
Surgical Oncology
Trauma Surgery
Urological Gynecology

Income Offered to Top 20 Recruited Specialties

(Base salary or income guarantee only, does not include production bonus or benefits)

	Low	Average	High
Family Practice			
2006/07	$120,000	$161,000	$250,000
2005/06	$115,000	$145,000	$220,000
2004/05	$125,000	$150,000	$200,000
2003/04	$120,000	$146,000	$195,000
Family Practice with Obstetrics			
2006/07	$145,000	$159,000	$200,000
2005/06	$140,000	$158,000	$180,000
2004/05	N/A	N/A	N/A
2003/04	N/A	N/A	N/A
Internal Medicine			
2006/07	$135,000	$174,000	$275,000
2005/06	$130,000	$162,000	$250,000
2004/05	$130,000	$161,000	$210,000
2003/04	$125,000	$152,000	$200,000
Hospitalist			
2006/07	$145,000	$180,000	$250,000
2005/06	$140,000	$175,000	$190,000
2004/05	$150,000	$171,000	$210,000
2003/04	$140,000	$162,000	$200,000
Radiology			
2006/07	$250,000	$380,000	$500,000
2005/06	$240,000	$351,000	$500,000
2004/05	$250,000	$355,000	$500,000
2003/04	$240,000	$336,000	$450,000
Orthopedic Surgery			
2006/07	$250,000	$413,000	$650,000
2005/06	$250,000	$370,000	$515,000
2004/05	$250,000	$361,000	$650,000
2003/04	$240,000	$330,000	$500,000
Cardiology			
2006/07	$250,000	$391,000	$500,000
2005/06	$175,000	$342,000	$500,000
2004/05	$234,000	$320,000	$525,000
2003/04	$230,000	$292,000	$500,000

	Low	Average	High
OB/GYN			
2006/07	$200,000	$247,000	$345,000
2005/06	$175,000	$234,000	$450,000
2004/05	$200,000	$247,000	$320,000
2003/04	$185,000	$242,000	$325,000
General Surgery			
2006/07	$225,000	$301,000	$350,000
2005/06	$150,000	$272,000	$350,000
2004/05	$220,000	$255,000	$310,000
2003/04	$210,000	$248,000	$300,000
Emergency Medicine			
2006/07	$150,000	$239,000	$300,000
2005/06	$130,000	$210,000	$270,000
2004/05	$140,000	$246,000	$270,000
2003/04	$120,000	$218,000	$260,000
Psychiatry			
2006/07	$160,000	$186,000	$230,000
2005/06	$130,000	$174,000	$230,000
2004/05	$140,000	$176,000	$250,000
2003/04	$130,000	$164,000	$260,000
Gastroenterology			
2006/07	$200,000	$365,000	$450,000
2005/06	$175,000	$315,000	$500,000
2004/05	$230,000	$298,000	$340,000
2003/04	$210,000	$250,000	$325,000
Urology			
2006/07	$275,000	$400,000	$500,000
2005/06	$250,000	$320,000	$375,000
2004/05	$250,000	$329,000	$340,000
2003/04	$220,000	$294,000	$325,000
Pediatrics			
2006/07	$115,000	$159,000	$200,000
2005/06	$115,000	$151,000	$180,000
2004/05	$110,000	$151,000	$180,000
2003/04	$110,000	$145,000	$170,000
CRNA			
2006/07	$130,000	$164,000	$200,000
2005/06	$87,000	$156,000	$210,000
2004/05	$75,000	$150,000	$190,000
2003/04	$70,000	$145,000	$190,000

Type of Guarantee (of 644 searches offering guarantees)

	Net Collections Guarantee	Gross Collections Guarantee
2006/07	501(78%)	143 (22%)
2005/06	736 (81%)	173 (19%)
2004/05	827 (88%)	113 (12%)
2003/04	916 (86%)	149 (14%)

Term of Guarantee (of 644 searches offering guarantees)

	1 Year	2 Year	3 Year
2006/07	411 (64%)	200 (31%)	33 (5%)
2005/06	591 (65%)	315 (35%)	3 (1%)
2004/05	708 (76%)	220 (23%)	8 (1%)
2003/04	852 (80%)	203 (19%)	10 (1%)

Searches Offering "Forgiveness" of Guarantee (of 644 searches offering guarantees)

	Forgiveness	No Forgiveness
2006/07	613 (95%)	31(5%)
2005/06	827 (91%)	82 (9%)
2004/05	884 (94%)	56 (6%)
2003/04	1,012 (95%)	53 (5%)

Time Period of Forgiveness (of 381 searches offering forgiveness)

	1 Year	2 Year	3 Year	Other / N/A
2006/07	24 (4%)	244 (40%)	308 (50%)	37 (6%)
2005/06	9 (1%)	298 (36%)	504 (61%)	16 (2%)
2004/05	38 (4%)	547 (58%)	303 (32%)	52 (6%)
2003/04	30 (3%)	516 (51%)	405 (40%)	61 (6%)

Paying Relocation

	Yes	No
2006/07	2,954 (98%)	62 (2%)
2005/06	2,815 (99%)	25 (1%)
2004/05	2,677 (99%)	10 (1%)
2003/04	2,578 (99%)	16 (1%)

Amount of Relocation Allowance

	Low	Average	High
2006/07	$1,000	$9,808	$75,000
2005/06	$3,000	$10,060	$20,000
2004/05	$3,500	$8,850	$20,000
2003/04	$2,000	$9,250	$22,000

Signing Bonus Offered

	Yes	No
2006/07	2,173 (72%)	843 (28%)
2005/06	1,650 (58%)	1190 (42%)
2004/05	1,236 (46%)	1,451 (54%)
2003/04	1,290 (50%)	1,304 (50%)

Amount of Bonus

	Low	Average	High
2006/07	$5,000	$20,000	$100,000
2005/06	$5,000	$20,480	$75,000
2004/05	$5,000	$14,030	$50,000
2003/04	$5,000	$15,500	$45,000

Paying Continuing Medical Education (CME)

	Yes	No
2006/07	2,746 (91%)	270 (9%)
2005/06	2,558 (90%)	282 (10%)
2004/05	2,498 (93%)	189 (7%)
2003/04	2,412 (93%)	182 (7%)

Amount of CME

	Low	Average	High
2006/07	$1,000	$3,312	$15,000
2005/06	$1,500	$3,830	$10,000
2004/05	$1,000	$3,350	$15,000
2003/04	$1,500	$3,250	$10,000

Paying Additional Benefits

	2006/07	2005/06	2004/05	2003/04
Health Insurance	91%	91%	92%	96%
Malpractice	91%	92%	93%	90%
Retirement	72%	70%	72%	70%
Disability	69%	70%	74%	70%
Educational Loan Forgiveness	26%	34%	14%	16%

TRENDS AND OBSERVATIONS

Merritt Hawkins & Associates **2007 Review of Physician Recruiting Incentives** underscores several trends in physician recruiting that have emerged over the last two to three years. Foremost among these is the reemergence of primary care, defined in this review as family practice, general internal medicine and pediatrics. Demand for these specialties peaked in the 1990s during the heyday of managed care, but has since declined, while demand for surgical and diagnostic specialists increased. In the mid-1990s, approximately 75 percent of Merritt Hawkins & Associates®' physician search assignments were for primary care physicians. By the early to mid part of this decade, this paradigm was reversed and about 75 percent of Merritt Hawkins & Associates search assignments were for surgical or diagnostic specialists.

The 2007 review indicates that hospitals, medical groups and other organizations have again shifted their recruiting emphasis toward primary care, even as demand for a variety of surgical and diagnostic specialists remains strong. In the 12-month period from April 1, 2006 to March 31, 2007, family practice and general internal medicine were Merritt Hawkins & Associates two most requested physician search assignments. Search assignments for pediatricians, which have been flat or declining for close to 10 years, also rose during this period. In addition, search assignments for obstetricians/gynecologists (who are considered primary care physicians by some observers) increased in the 2006/07 review period, after several years of flat or declining growth.

The graph below illustrates percent of growth in primary care search assignments from 2003/04 to 2006/07.

Growth in Primary Care Searches / 2003/04 – 2006/07

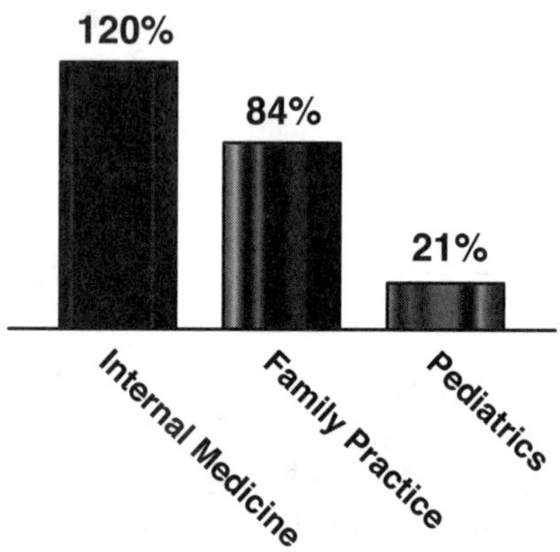

Primary care is enjoying a comeback for several reasons. In the 1990s, many medical school graduates gravitated toward primary care residencies, creating a bulge in supply, while medical graduates are largely avoiding primary care today. Many residency programs, particularly in family practice, fall short of filling their available positions. This dip in supply coincides with a renewed focus that hospitals and medical groups are putting on primary care after several years of neglect. In the case of internal medicine, population aging is driving demand, as is a general shortage of internal medicine sub-specialists. Unable to find an adequate number of gastroenterologists, cardiologists and other IM sub-specialists, some facilities are recruiting general internists to pick up the slack.

The strong comeback of primary care does not necessarily indicate that interest in specialty areas is declining. The 2007 review shows a drop in demand for radiologists, cardiologists, general surgeons and orthopedic surgeons relative to the previous three years. However, relative to the early parts of this decade and to the 1990s, demand for these specialists remains high. The 2007 review does indicate a significant decline in demand for specialists in anesthesiology, reflected in the reduced number of search assignments for both anesthesiologists and certified registered nurse anesthetists (CRNAs) during the 2006/07 review period. This decline in search assignments is likely a result of the increased number of specialists being trained in these areas, which has created a closer balance between supply and demand, rather than a decline in procedures requiring anesthesia.

By contrast, demand is up significantly for hospitalists who provide inpatient care in a hospital setting. Hospitalists are proving a popular and effective way of enhancing quality of care, reducing medical errors and managing costs. In addition, by relieving office-based physicians of inpatient work, hospitalists can increase medical staff retention and satisfaction rates. However, because so many internal medicine practitioners are choosing to practice as hospitalists, the supply of general internists has become constrained. At the same time, the growing number of older patients is creating more demand for general internists, making this one of the most difficult search assignments to fill today.

While demand for physicians in various specialties tends to run in cycles, the general trend in physician recruiting today is characterized by a strong demand for physicians in all specialties virtually across the board, coupled with a limited supply. The nation continues to face a physician shortage, which is discussed in greater detail in the Merritt Hawkins & Associates book, *Will the Last Physician in America Please Turn Off the Lights?*

MORE HOSPITALS EMPLOYING PHYSICIANS

The 2007 review also confirms another physician recruiting pattern that has become apparent over the last three years: An increasing number of hospitals are employing physicians. Direct employment of physicians by hospitals was one hallmark of managed care in the 1990s, but the practice was largely dropped as hospitals found the physician employment model problematic. The 2007 review shows that 43 percent of the Merritt Hawkins & Associates 2006/07 physician search assignments were for hospital settings, up significantly from 23 percent in 2005/06 and from 19 percent in 2004/05.

The graph below shows those Merritt Hawkins & Associates search assignments that featured hospital settings over the last five years.

Hospital-Based Search Assignments

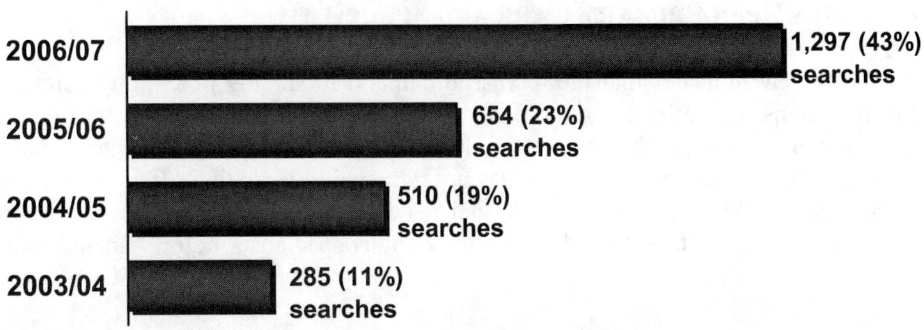

The new trend toward hospital employment of physicians is different from the 1990s, when hospitals approached physicians about employment opportunities rather than the reverse. Today many physicians, specialists in particular, are seeking hospital employment to relieve them of the stress of high malpractice rates, the struggle for reimbursement, administrative duties and the general risks and hassles of private practice. Hospital employment is viewed favorably by many physicians today and, in our experience, hospitals offering employed positions may enjoy an advantage over those that do not. In addition, Stark laws pertaining to physician recruitment can create scenarios where it is more practical for hospitals to employ physicians than to assist them in establishing independent practices.

The increase in employed positions is also reflected in the types of financial offers made to physicians. Salaries were offered in 79 percent of all Merritt Hawkins & Associates search assignments during the 2006/07 review period, compared to 68 percent in 2004/05 and 59 percent in 2002/04. Only 21 percent of searches offered income guarantees, which typically are offered to physicians in independent (non-employed) practice settings.

Geographic Recruiting Patterns

The 2007 review indicates that Merritt Hawkins & Associates represented physician search assignments in 48 states (all states except Hawaii and Delaware) during the review period. Hospitals, medical groups and other organizations in almost every state found it necessary or desirable to retain the services of physician search firms such as Merritt Hawkins & Associates suggesting that physician recruitment challenges exist nationwide, even in states with high physician-to-population ratios such as Massachusetts and New York.

The general shortage of physicians is also underlined by the fact that the plurality of the searches Merritt Hawkins & Associates conducted in 2006/07 (40 percent) were located in cities of 100,000 or more. Medical organizations in communities of all sizes now require the services of physidan search firms such as Merritt Hawkins & Associates suggesting that physician shortages are not localized to rural areas.

Incentives Up in Primary Care and Specialties

The 2007 review indicates that the increased demand for family practitioners, internists and pediatricians was reflected in the financial incentives offered to recruit them. While demand for primary care physicians (family physicians and internists in particular) has increased in the last several years, this was not reflected in recruiting offers made to them until this year. In Merritt Hawkins & Associates experience, it often takes the market a year or two to adjust to rising demand for certain specialists before financial offers increase.

Average salary or income-guarantee offers ma de to family practitioners increased from $145,000 in 2005/06 to $161,000 in 2006/07, a gain of 11 percent, while average offers made to general internists increased from $162,000 in 2005/06 to $174,000 in 2006/07, a gain of 7 percent. Other specialists also saw significant gains in average financial offers, including radiologists, orthopedic surgeons, cardiologists, general surgeons, gastroenterologists, urologists, otolaryngologists and neurosurgeons. These gains suggest a continued high demand for physicians in a wide range of specialties. Anesthesiology was the only specialty tracked by the review that showed a decline. The graph below shows the medical specialties that had the greatest increases in income offers during the 2006/2007 review period.

Specialties Showing Highest Gain in Base Income Offers/2005/06 – 2006/07

	Base Income 2005/06	Base Income 2006/07	% Increase
Urology	$320,000	$400,000	25%
Otolaryngology	$272,000	$312,000	15%
Cardiology	$342,000	$391,000	14%
Emergency Medicine	$210,000	$239,000	14%
Orthopedic Surgery	$370,000	$413,000	12%
Family Practice	$145,000	$161,000	11%

SIGNING BONUSES NOW STANDARD

The number of hospitals, medical groups and other organizations offering physicians signing bonuses has steadily increased over the last 10 years, in Merritt Hawkins & Associates' experience. In the 1990s, searches offering signing bonuses were the exception; the 2007 review indicates that they are now generally the rule. Signing bonuses were offered in 72 percent of the recruiting assignments Merritt Hawkins & Associates conducted in 2006/07, up from 58 percent in 2005/06, 46 percent in 2004/05 and 50 percent in 2003/04.

The graph below illustrates the increase in the use of signing bonuses over the last several years

Searches Offering Signing Bonuses

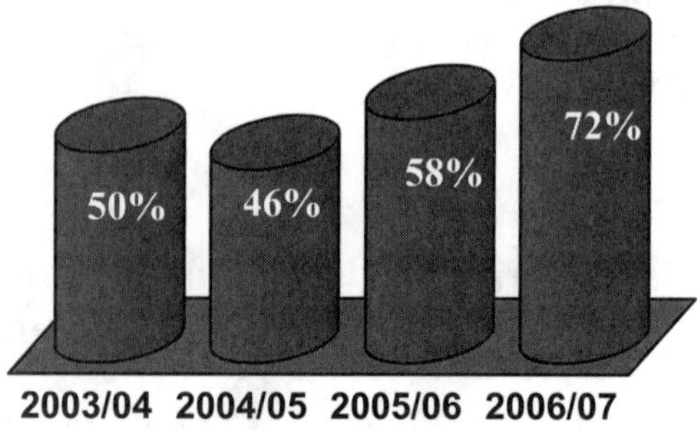

Signing bonuses offered in 2006/07 averaged $20,000, roughly the same as 2005/06, though an increase from $14,000 in 2004/05 and from $15,500 in 2003/04.

Certain other incentives, such as paid relocation, paid continuing medical education (CME), health and malpractice insurance are standard in the majority of Merritt Hawkins & Associates physician search assignments. The average relocation allowance offered in 2006/07 was $9,808, about the same as the previous year, while the average CME allowance was $3,312 also about the same as the previous year.

SUMMARY

Merritt Hawkins & Associates 2007 Review of Physician Recruiting Incentives underscores the fact that the demand for primary care physicians continues to grow while demand for most specialists remains strong. Hospital employment of physicians also appears to be increasing as many physicians seek the security and relative simplicity of an employed position. Financial incentives offered to recruit physicians generally are up, while the use of signing bonuses has increased. The 2007 review also indicates that physician recruitment is a national challenge, as Merritt Hawkins & Associates conducted search assignments in virtually all 50 states in 2006/07.

The MHA Group® / Additional Surveys

Merritt Hawkins & Associates is a division of AMN Healthcare, the nation's largest health care staffing firm. Other surveys conducted by Merritt Hawkins & Associates or other AMN brands include

- Survey of Physicians 50 to 65 Years Old
- Physician Inpatient / Outpatient Revenue Survey
- Survey of Final Year Medical Residents
- Hospital Physician Recruitment Trends Survey
- Survey of Primary Care Physicians
- Review of Temporary Health Care Staffing Trends & Incentives
- Review of Temporary Health Care Staffing Trends & Incentives (Mid-level Providers)
- Survey of Hospital Chief Nursing Officers
- Survey of Male Nurses
- Survey of Travel Nurses
- Survey of Nurse Students

Books written by Merritt Hawkins & Associates' executives:

Will the Last Physician in America Please Turn Off the Lights?
A Look at America's Looming Physician Shortage
© 2004 Merritt Hawkins & Associates®

Merritt Hawkins & Associates® Guide to Physician Recruiting
© 2007 Merrit Hawkins & Associates®

To order these books from the publisher, visit www.practicesupport.com.

Merritt Hawkins & Associates®

2007 Physician Inpatient/Outpatient Revenue Survey

INTRODUCTION:

Merritt Hawkins & Associates is a national physician search and consulting firm specializing in the recruitment of physicians in all medical specialties. Established in 1987, Merritt Hawkins & Associates is a division of AMN Healthcare, the largest health care staffing organization in the United States.

As part of our effort to monitor trends in health care staffing, we conduct an ongoing series of surveys covering a range of staffing issues, including physician recruiting incentives, physician practice patterns, hospital recruiting patterns, and related topics. This report summarizes Merritt Hawkins & Associates' third survey of the revenue physicians in various specialties generate for their affiliated hospitals. This periodic survey was conducted previously by Merritt Hawkins & Associates in 2002 and in 2004.

The survey is intended to provide benchmark data hospitals can use to develop a "quantitative analysis" of their physician recruiting programs. A quantitative analysis as defined by the U.S. Internal Revenue Service (IRS) establishes the financial benefits that newly recruited physicians will bring to a hospital. These benefits may support the hospital's mission of providing quality care to the community by creating revenue streams necessary to its continued or its enhanced operation. A quantitative analysis therefore may serve as part of a hospital's physician recruiting plan by demonstrating the financial benefits to the hospital of physician recruitment. It should be noted, however, that a physician recruiting plan also should include a "qualitative analysis" demonstrating how newly recruited physicians will enhance quality of care in the community.

Survey data also may be used in setting physician compensation levels or recruiting incentives through a cost/benefit analysis comparing the aggregate expense of recruiting physicians to the average revenue generated by physicians in various specialties.

METHODOLOGY

Merritt Hawkins & Associates mailed the Physician Inpatient/Outpatient Revenue Survey to 5,000 hospital chief financial officers (CFOs) nationwide. The survey form was mailed once in October, 2006 and again in February, 2007. The survey could be taken anonymously or those CFOs requesting survey results could identify themselves and their facilities. The survey asked hospital CFOs to indicate the combined ***net*** inpatient and outpatient revenue generated annually for their facilities by a single, full time equivalent (FTE) physician in a variety of specialties. In the case of primary care physicians (defined as family practitioners, general internists, and pediatricians), survey respondents were asked to determine revenue from direct admissions, lab tests, etc., not indirect revenue primary care physicians may have generated from patient referrals to specialists utilizing the hospital.

The survey provided various revenue ranges and allowed CFOs to select the most appropriate range for each specialty. In lieu of indicating a range, CFOs also had the option of indicating on the survey form the specific amount of revenue generated annually for their hospital per a single physician in various specialties.

In cases where a range was indicated, the survey takes the midpoint of this range to determine a weighted average for each specialty. A total of 119 completed surveys were received. It should be noted that the volume of categorical responses varied by specialty. Not all returned survey forms included data for all specialties. In addition, the survey was self-selecting. Given these factors, figures for average revenue generated per medical specialty cannot be expected to reflect the experiences of all hospitals.

RESPONDING HOSPITALS BY NUMBER OF BEDS

Questionnaires were mailed to 5,000 chief financial officers (CFOs) at acute care hospitals throughout the country, once in October, 2006 and once in February, 2007. Responding hospitals by number of beds are indicated below, with comparisons to the surveys conducted in 2002 and 2004.

2002

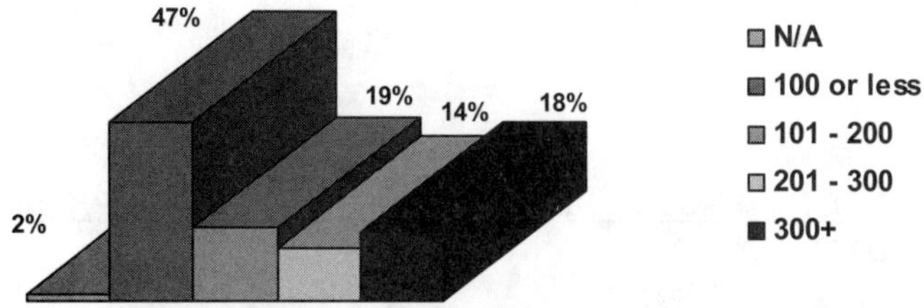

2004

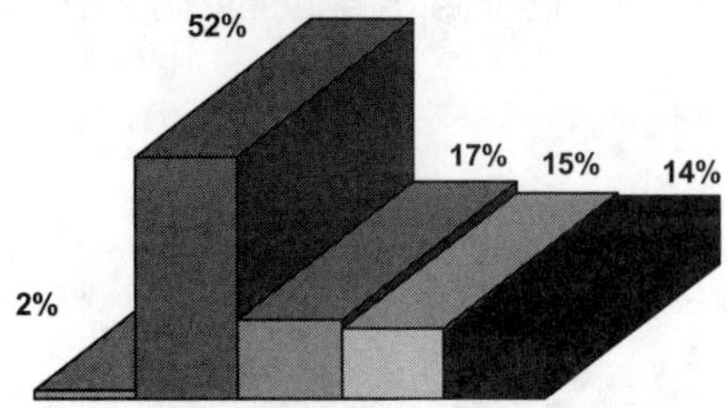

2007

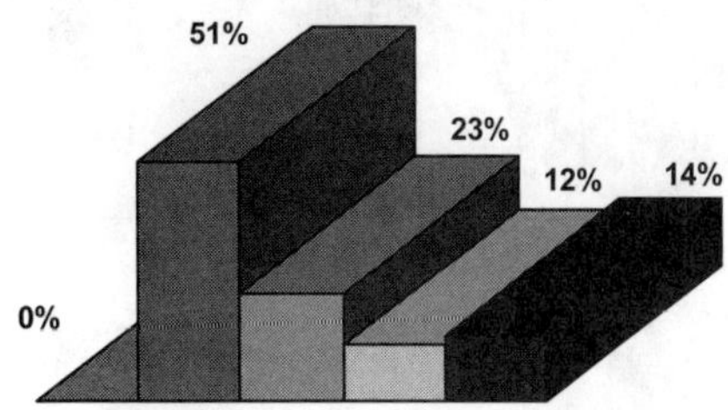

RESPONDING HOSPITALS BY NUMBER OF BEDS (YEAR TO YEAR COMPARISON)

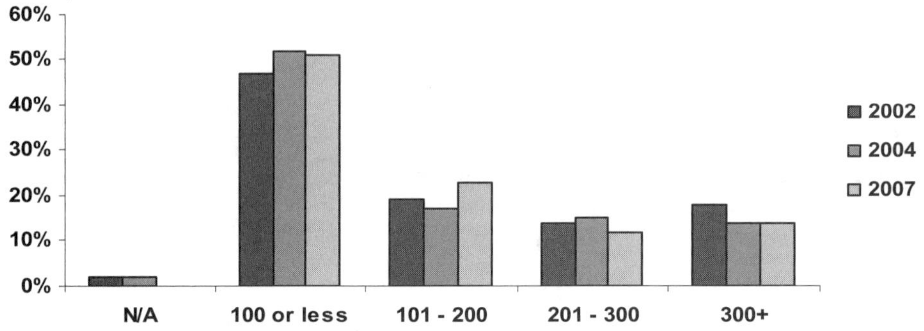

AVERAGE REVENUE GENERATED BY PRIMARY CARE PHYSICIANS, SPECIALISTS, AND ALL PHYSICIANS

(Primary care is defined in this survey as family practice, general internal medicine, and pediatrics. 2007 numbers for "Specialties" and "All Specialties" include average revenue generated by ophthalmologists, a specialty not included in the 2002 and 2004 surveys)

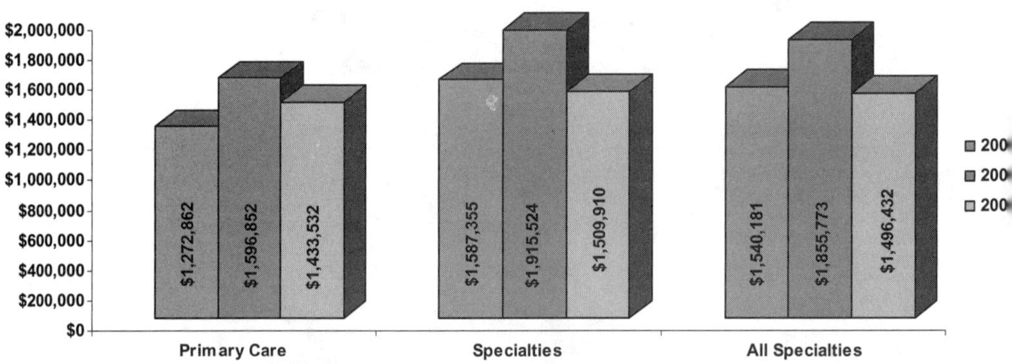

REVENUE GENERATED BY SPECIALTY

The graph below indicates average annual inpatient/outpatient revenue generated for hospitals by physicians in various medical specialties.

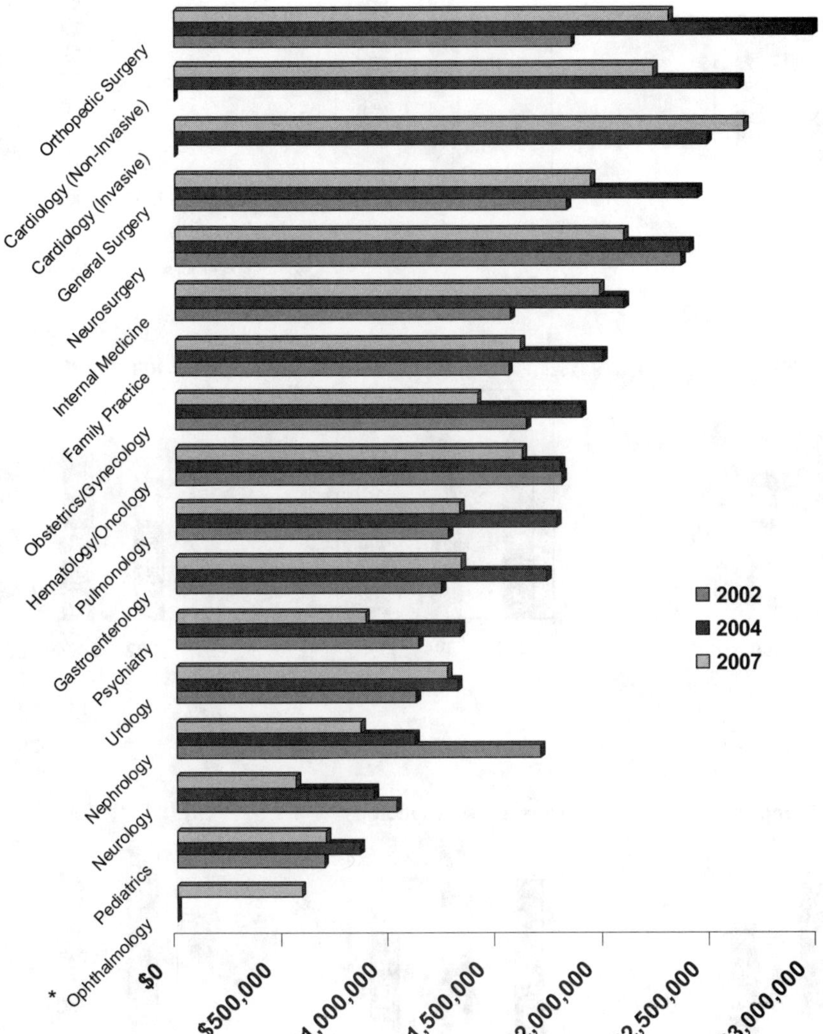

*Ophthalmology included for the first time in 2007

SPECIALTY REVENUE COMPARISION

Average annual inpatient/outpatient revenue generated by physicians for their affiliated hospitals by specialty, 2007 figures compared to 2004 and 2002

Orthopedic Surgery

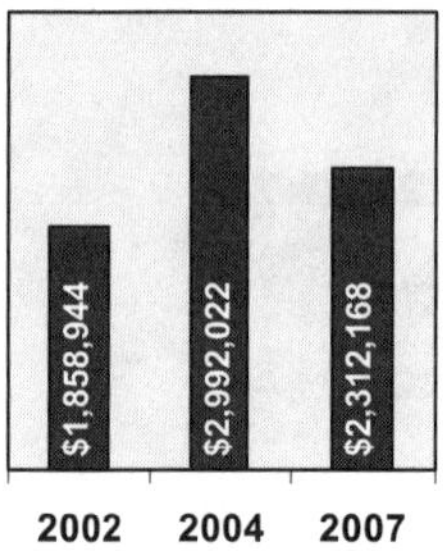

Cardiology (Non-Invasive)*

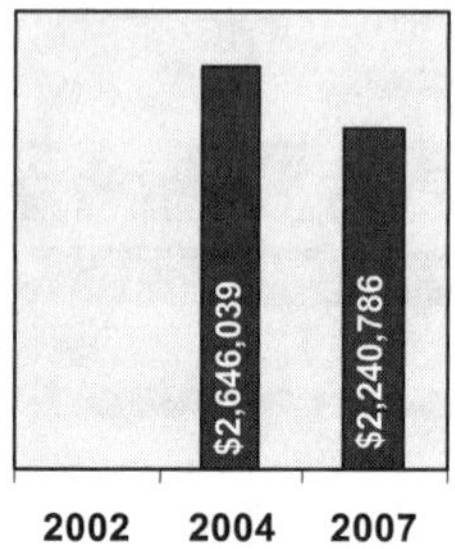

Cardiology (Invasive)*

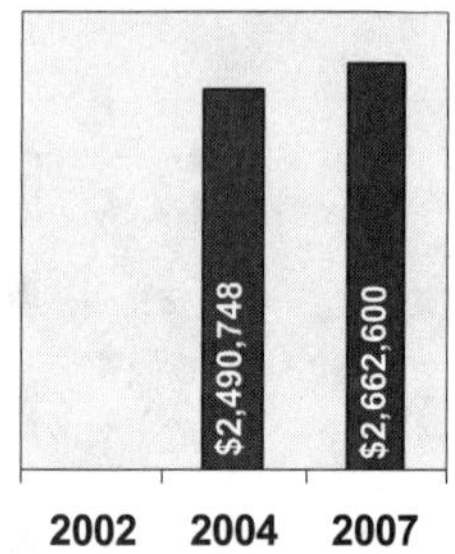

*Invasive and Non-Invasive Cardiology were not surveyed independently in 2002

General Surgery

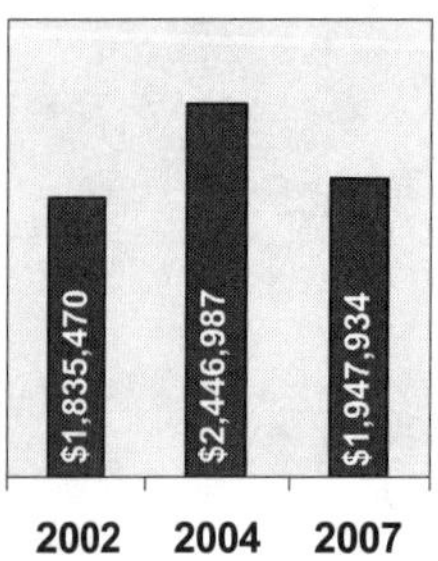

Neurosurgery

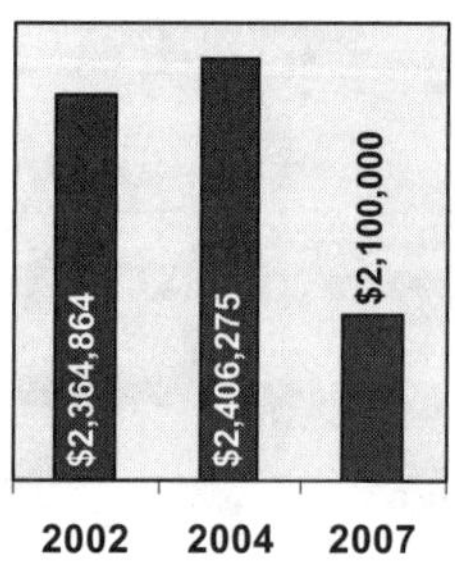

Internal Medicine

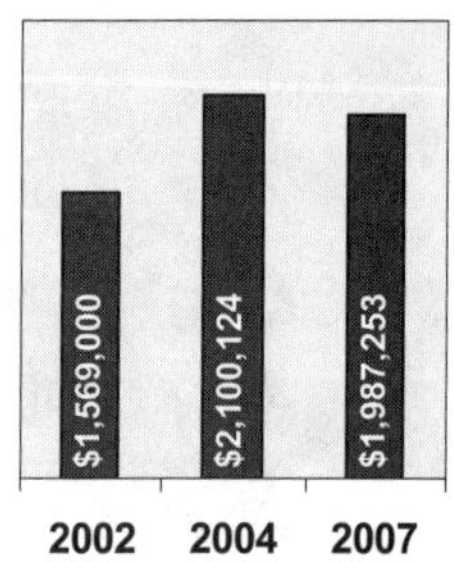

Family Practice

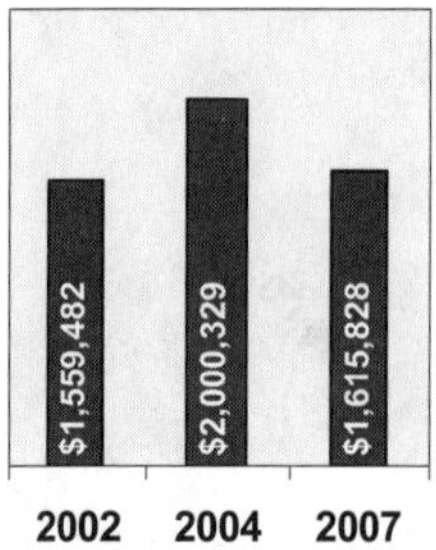

Obstetrics/Gynecology

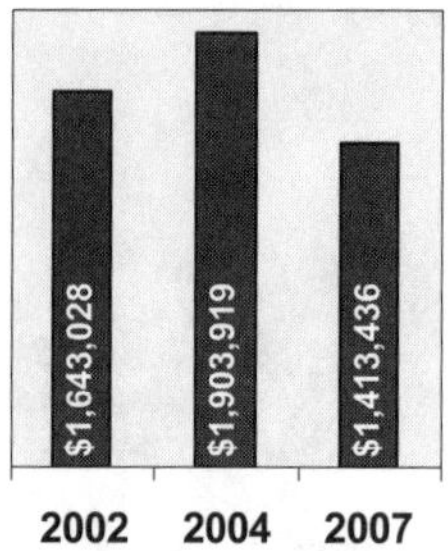

Hematology/Oncology

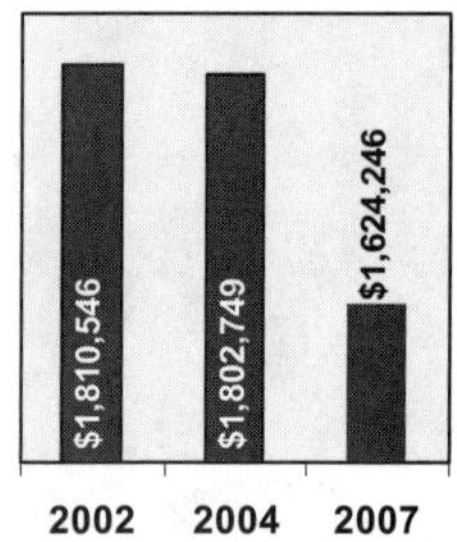

Pulmonology

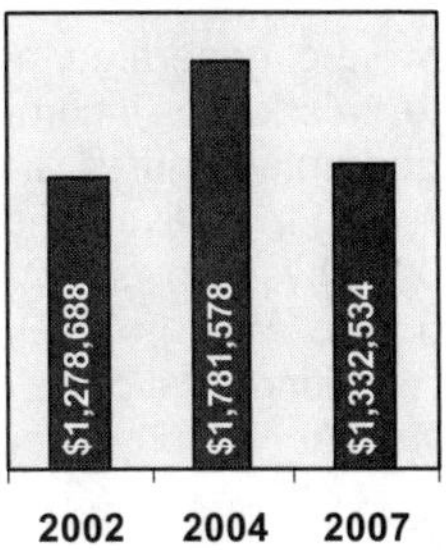

Gastroenterology

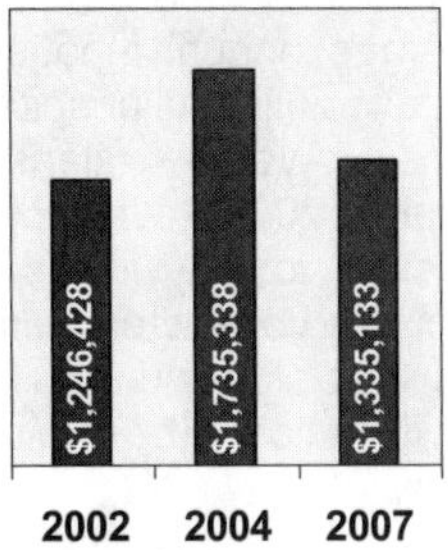

Psychiatry

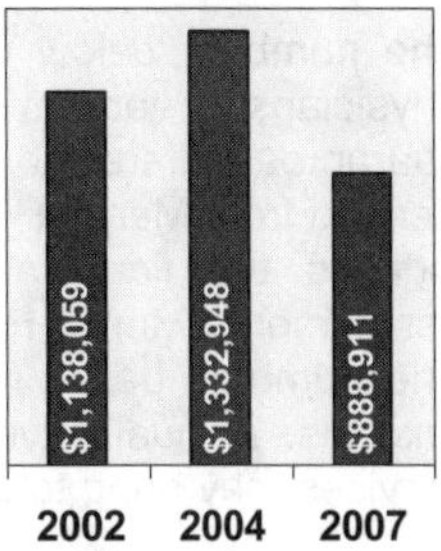

Urology

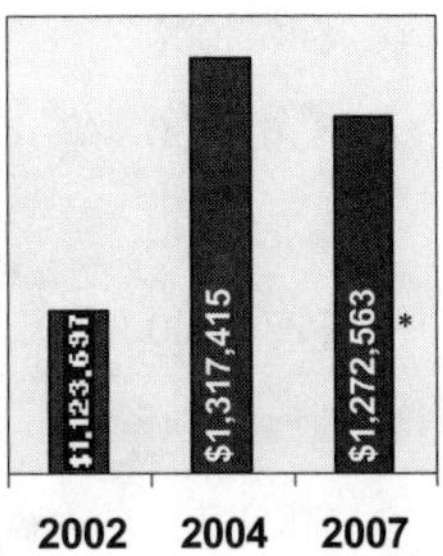

Nephrology

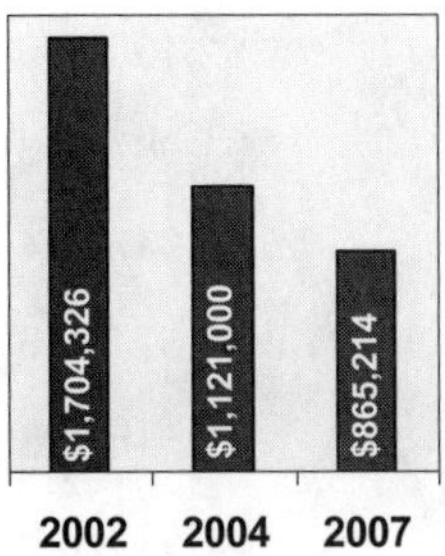

Neurology

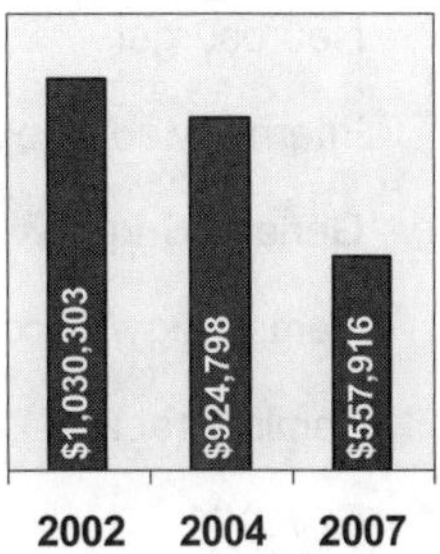

Pediatrics

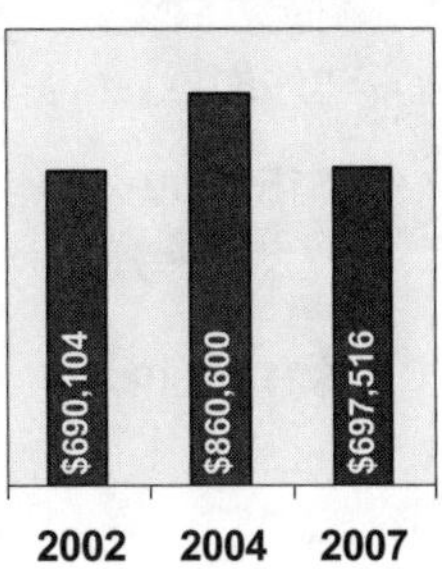

Ophthalmology *

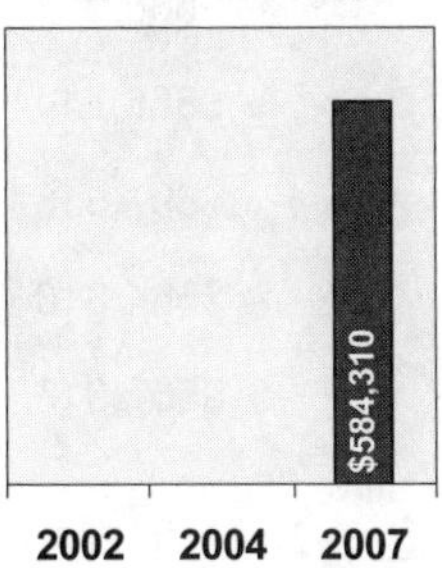

*Ophthalmology not included in 2002/2004

COST/BENEFIT ANALYSIS

The numbers below contrast the average annual inpatient/outpatient revenue generated by physicians in various specialties for their affiliated hospitals with average salaries or income guarantees offered to recruit physicians. Average salaries and income guarantee figures are derived from Merritt Hawkins & Associates' 2006 Review of Physician Recruiting Incentives and indicate the financial incentives offered to physicians in some 2,800 physician search assignments Merritt Hawkins & Associates conducted from March 31, 2005 to April 1, 2006. The numbers below may be used as part of a "quantitative" physician recruiting cost/benefit analysis. A "qualitative" analysis also will factor in the quality of care benefits that new physician services may bring to a given community.

Specialty	Revenue	Avg. Starting Salary*
Cardiology (Invasive)	$2,662,600	$342,000
Orthopedic Surgery	$2,312,168	$370,000
Cardiology/Non-Inv.	$2,240,786	$342,000
Neurosurgery	$2,100,000	$489,000
Internal Medicine	$1,987,253	$162,000
General Surgery	$1,947,934	$272,000
Hematology/Oncology	$1,624,246	$275,000
Family Practice	$1,615,828	$145,000
OB/GYN	$1,413,436	$234,000
Gastroenterology	$1,335,133	$315,000
Pulmonology	$1,332,534	$248,000
Urology	$1,272,563	$320,000
Psychiatry	$888,911	$174,000
Nephrology	$865,214	$225,000
Pediatrics	$697,516	$151,000
Ophthalmology	$584,310	N/A
Neurology	$557,916	$210,000

*2006 MHA Recruitment Incentives Survey

TRENDS AND OBSERVATIONS

Merritt Hawkins & Associates' 2007 Physician Inpatient/Outpatient Revenue Survey marks the third time we have collected data regarding the net revenue physicians in various specialties generate for their affiliated hospitals through patient referrals, admissions, treatments and procedures.

The 2007 Survey indicates that average net inpatient/outpatient revenue generated by physicians for their affiliated hospitals decreased by specialty relative to 2004 in most cases. Average revenue generated by primary care physicians declined from $1,596,852 in 2004 to $1,433,532 in 2007. However, revenue generated by primary care physicians in 2007 was up compared to the 2002 figure ($1,272,862).

Average revenue generated by specialist physicians declined from $1,915,524 in 2004 to $1,509,910 in 2007. Revenue generated by medical specialists in 2007 also was down compared to the 2002 figure ($1,587,355). A partial explanation for this is that ophthalmology, a specialty that generates relatively little revenue for most hospitals, was included in the survey for the first time in 2007, bringing down the overall average for specialists and for all physicians (primary care and specialists.)

Average revenue generated by all physicians, primary care and specialists, declined from $1,855,773 in 2004 to $1,496,432 in 2007. Revenue generated by all physicians also was down compared to the 2002 figure ($1,540,181).

The survey did not ask respondents to provide any reasons for increases or decreases in annual revenue generated for their hospitals by physicians. It is possible that hospitals surveyed in 2007 may be seeing fewer patient admissions or experiencing declines in reimbursement for treatments and procedures. In some cases, hospitals may be losing well reimbursing elective and other procedures to free standing surgery centers and other competitors

Despite relative declines, the survey indicates that physicians continue to generate a significant level of revenue for their affiliated hospitals, close to $1.5 million on average per physician. As the drivers of admissions, tests, and procedures, physicians are essential to the economic well being of hospitals and also are critical to the quality of care hospitals provide for their communities.

Staff Care®

The Leader in Locum Tenens Staffing

Member of the National Association of Locum Tenens Organizations NALTO

Summary Report
2006 Review of Temporary Physician Staffing Trends

Overview

Staff Care is a national physician staffing firm specializing in matching temporary (i.e., *locum tenens)* physicians in all specialties with hospitals, medical groups, government facilities and other health care organizations requiring temporary physician services. Staff Care is a division of AMN Healthcare, the nation's largest health care staffing organization.

This report marks Staff Care's fourth Review of Temporary Physician Staffing Trends. The purpose of the Review is to quantify trends in temporary physician staffing and to provide benchmark data that may be useful to health care professionals and others who monitor developments in the health care staffing industry.

Methodology

The 2006 Review is based on telephone surveys conducted by Staff Care marketing and recruiting professionals and on a review of the firm's 2005 temporary staffing assignments.

Part I of the Review examines trends among the users of temporary physician services, including traditional acute care hospitals, medical groups, and state-supported facilities such as behavioral health centers and correctional facilities.

Part II of the Review examines trends among physicians working on a temporary (*locum tenens)* basis, including how they select opportunities, how they are perceived by colleagues, etc.

Part III of the survey is a review of the temporary physician staffing assignments Staff Care conducted in calendar year 2005. The breakdown of assignments by specialty, location and other factors is offered as an indicator of current physician supply and demand trends in *locum tenens.* Part III includes estimates of the current size of the temporary physician staffing market based on an extrapolation of Staff Care's market share of the industry.

The telephone surveys were conducted over the three month period from February 1, 2006 to April 30, 2006. Respondents were self-selected and included both Staff Care clients and non-clients and both physicians who have been matched to assignments by Staff Care and those who have not.

Survey of Users of Temporary Physician Staffing Services

Number of Surveys Completed = 662

Types of Facilities

Acute care hospitals...65%
Medical Groups...24%
Government facilities (correctional, behavioral, military)......9%
Other..2%

Questions Asked and Responses Received

Have you used locum tenens physicians any time in the last 12 months?

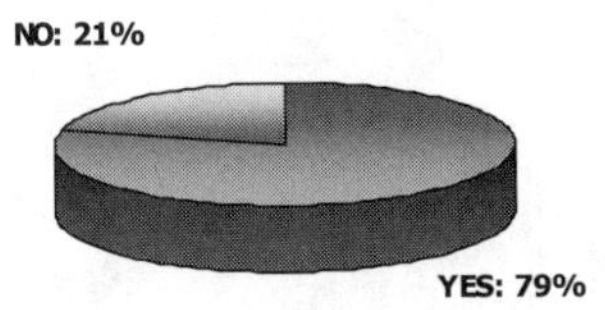

Currently Looking for Locum Tenens Physicians?

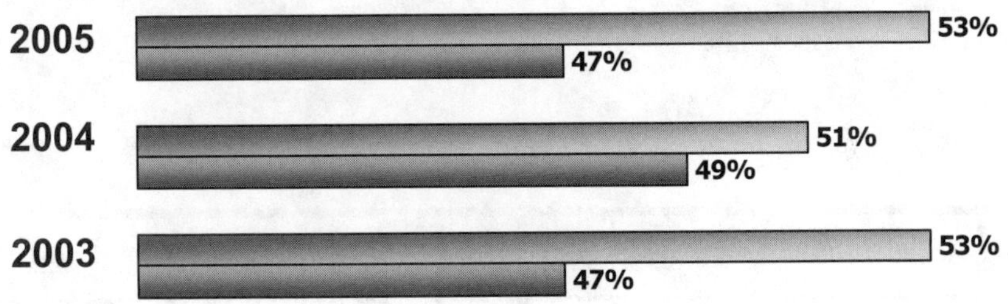

The Process Compared To Past Years

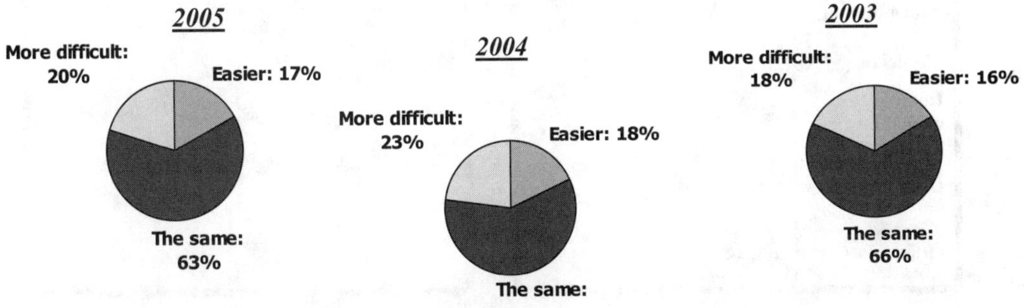

In a typical month, how many locum tenens physicians do you use?

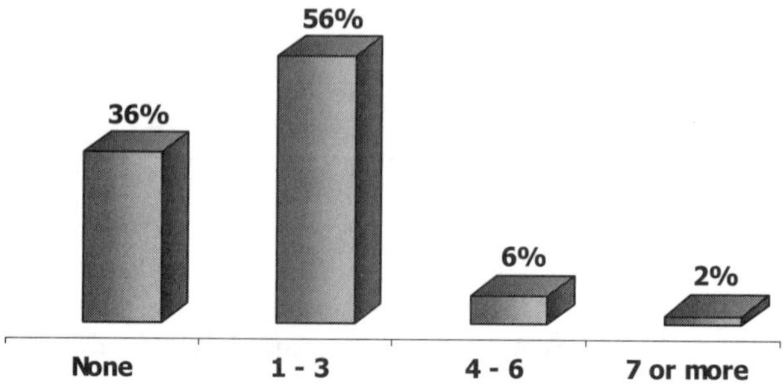

Why Use Locum Tenens?

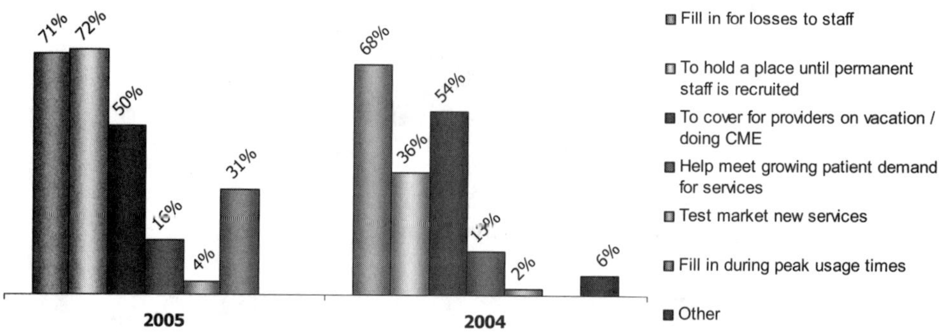

Benefits of Locum Tenens

PROs:	2005	2004	2003	2002
Prevent loss of revenue	43%	44%	36%	38%
Maintain continuity of care	70%	76%	72%	74%
Prevent "burn-out" of staff physicians	39%	27%	27%	16%
Immediate availability	54%	44%	44%	40%
Cost	4%	4%	2%	1%
Other	4%	5%	7%	1%

CONs:	2005	2004	2003	2002
Cost	81%	82%	80%	74%
Unfamiliar with practice	52%	45%	49%	48%
Learning curve with equipment and procedures	22%	22%	n/a	n/a
Other	28%	12%	4%	7%

What is YOUR perception of the skill level of locum tenens physicians?

Locums vs. Existing Staff

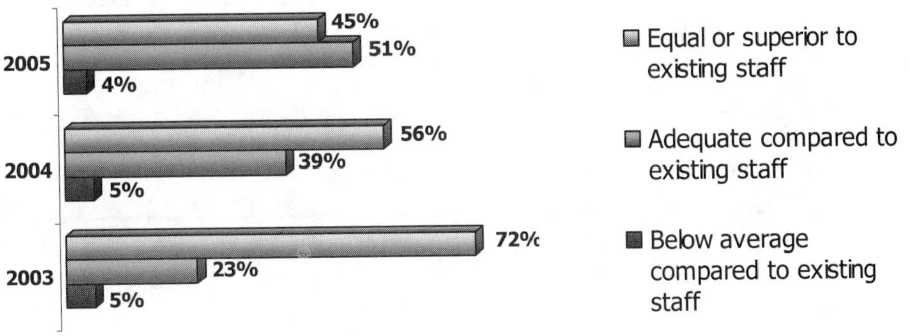

At *your* facility, how are locum tenens providers viewed by.

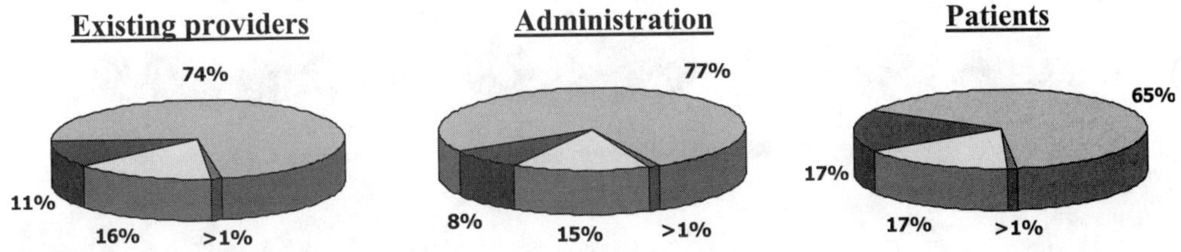

During The Search

How many temporary staffing firms do you generally work with?

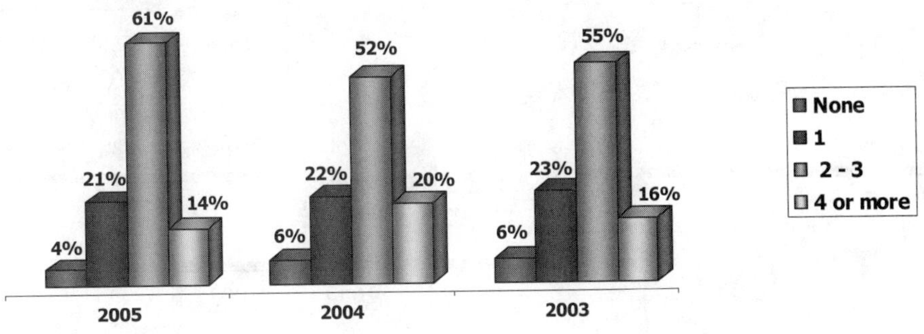

What is the most important factor in selecting a temporary staffing firm?

	2005*	2004	2003*	2002*	2001*
Quality of candidates presented	**69%**	37%	61%	58%	43%
Cost	**48%**	19%	39%	45%	30%
Promptness/availability of candidate	**70%**	32%	53%	49%	36%
Customer service	**39%**	7%	26%	21%	16%
Malpractice insurance	**16%**	1%	10%	23%	1%
Contract flexibility	**21%**	2%	8%	12%	9%
Other	**3%**	3%	3%	3%	7%

**Multiple responses possible in 2005, 2003, 2002, 2001*

Are they worth the cost?

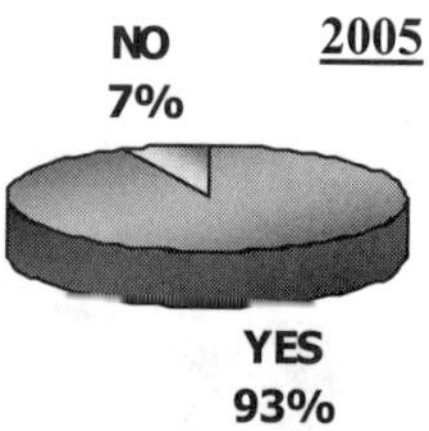

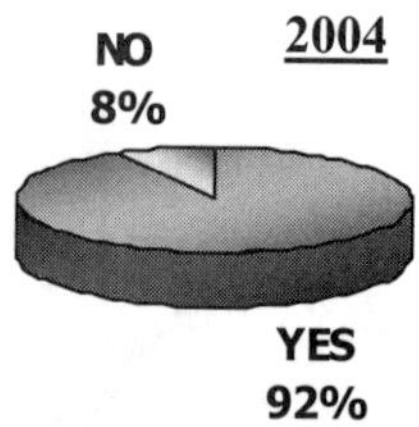

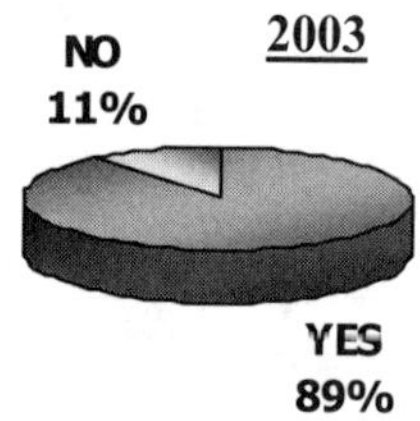

Compared to your staff physicians

How do Locum Tenens Physicians Stack Up?

Patients treated per day

	2005	2004	2003
More	2%	5%	2%
Fewer	34%	26%	30%
Same	64%	69%	68%

Time spent with patients

	2005	2004	2003
More	15%	10%	15%
Less	12%	11%	6%
Same	73%	79%	79%

Gross charges generated per day

	2005	2004	2003
More	2%	3%	2%
Fewer	37%	27%	26%
Same	61%	70%	72%

Trends and Observations

Part I of the Review suggests several trends among the users of *locum tenens* physician services, including managers or personnel directors at hospitals, medical groups, and government supported health facilities.

The survey indicates that about half of hospitals, medical groups and government supported health facilities are seeking locum tenens physicians at any one time. Forty-seven percent of those surveyed indicated that they are currently seeking *locum tenens* physicians to supplement their existing staffs, about the same percentage as in 2004 and the same percentage as in 2003. It sugggests that the need for locum tenens physicians is widespread and has been so for several years.

The process of finding locum tenens physicians became more difficult in 2005 than in 2004 for 23% of those surveyed, but easier for 18%. Over the last three years the majority of respondents have indicated that the process of finding locum tenens physicians has neither become more difficult nor easier relative to the previous year. With some exceptions, therefore, the supply of locum tenens physicians appears to be keeping pace with demand.

Use of locum tenens physicians among those surveyed varies. About one-third do not use a locum tenens physician in a typical month, while the majority (56%) use at least one. A minority (8%) use four or more.

Reasons those surveyed give for using locum tenens physicians also varies. The number who use locum tenens physicians to hold a place until a permanent physician is recruited increased from 36% in 2004 to 72% in 2005. This would seem to underscore the growing shortage of physicians nationally and the increasing role of temporary physicians as a staffing "stop gap."

Seventy-one percent of those surveyed indicated they use locum tenens physicians to fill in for losses to staff. Due to physician aging and the increased mobility of doctors, it is believed that losses to medical staffs are becoming more common, further driving the need for temporary physicians. Half of those surveyed (50%) indicated that they use locum tenens physicians to cover for providers on vacation/CME. A "controllable lifestyle" has become increasingly important to physicians, and many are seeking more regular vacation time than doctors were accustomed to in the past. This creates gaps in the medical staff, which many facilities may use locum tenens physicians to fill.

The main benefit of using locum tenens physicians, cited by 70% of those surveyed, is to maintain continuity of care. Cost was more frequently cited as a drawback to using locum tenens than any other factor. However, 93% of those surveyed indicated that locum tenens physicians are "worth the cost," up from 92% in 2004 and 89% in 2003.

Survey of Physicians Working On A Locum Tenens Basis

Number of Providers Surveyed = 735

Types of Providers
Primary care (family practice, internal medicine, pediatrics)…40%
Surgical / diagnostic specialists……………..……….…………….38%
Behavioral health…………………………………………..……….15%
Other……………………………………………………………..…….7%

Questions Asked and Responses Received

How Many Years As A Physician?

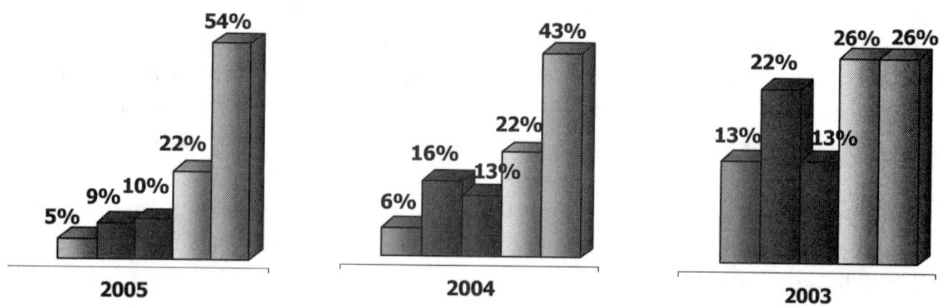

Locum Tenens Experience

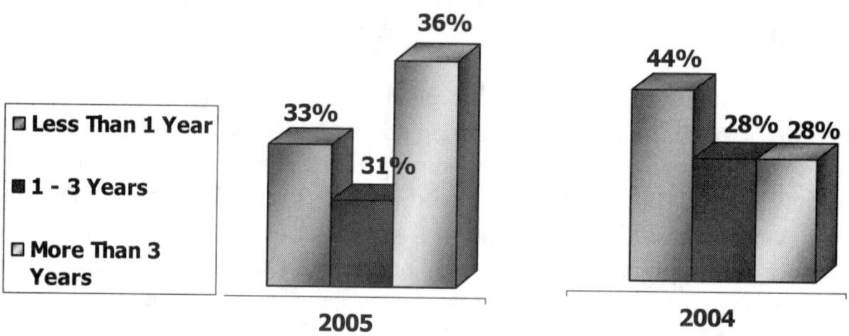

Number of Assignments / Assignment Length

Locum Tenens Assignments Worked Per Year

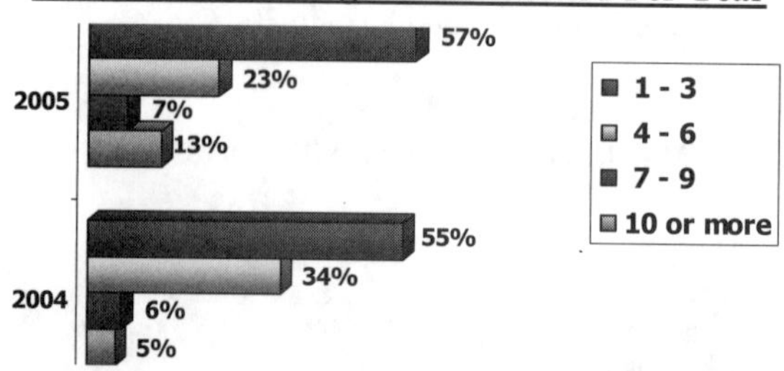

Ideal Assignment Length

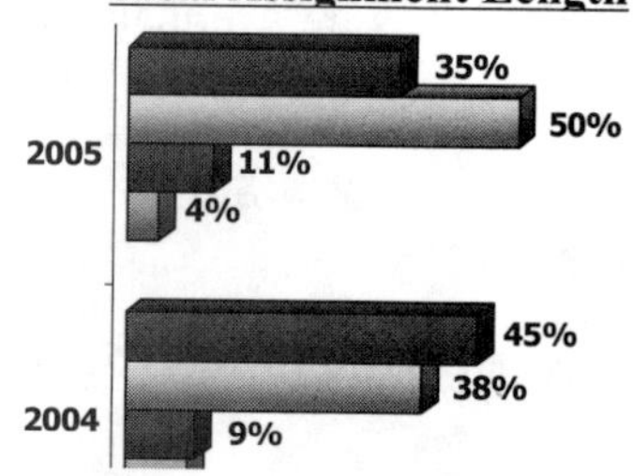

How long do you intend to practice on a temporary basis?

	2005	2004	2003	2002	2001
Until I find a permanent position	**18%**	18%	28%	30%	33%
Less than 1 year	**6%**	6%	8%	9%	25%
1 - 3 years	**25%**	33%	25%	35%	20%
More than 3 years	**51%**	43%	39%	26%	22%

Are You In a Permanent Position?

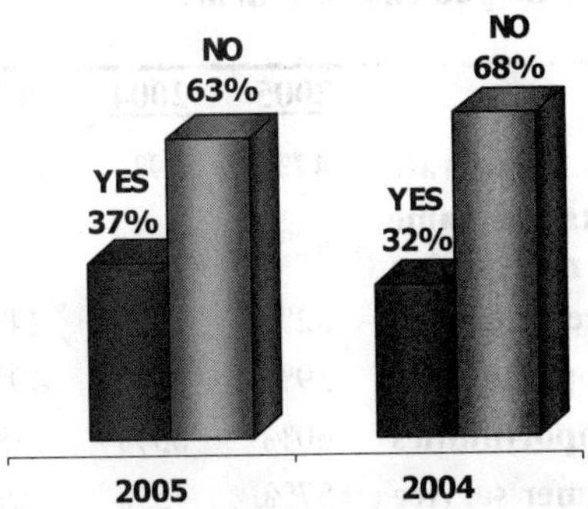

Are You looking For Perm?

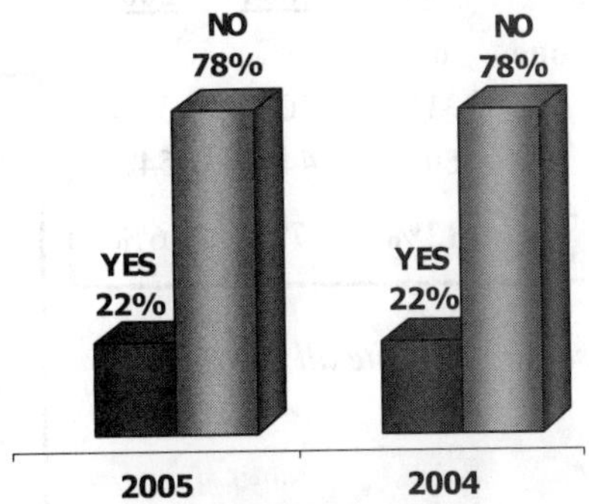

Have you ever worked in a permanent position?

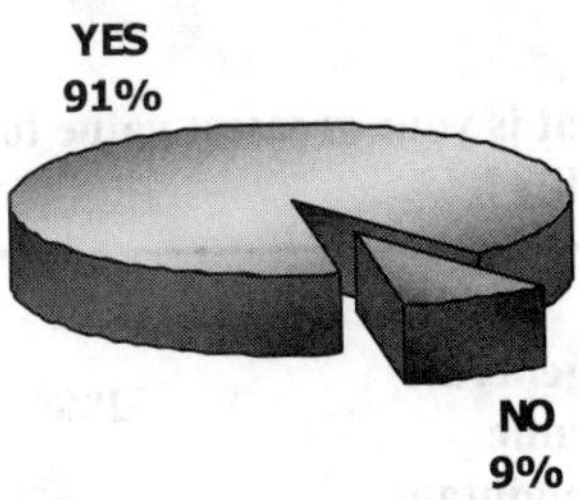

If yes, rate working as a locum tenens physician vs. working in a permanent position

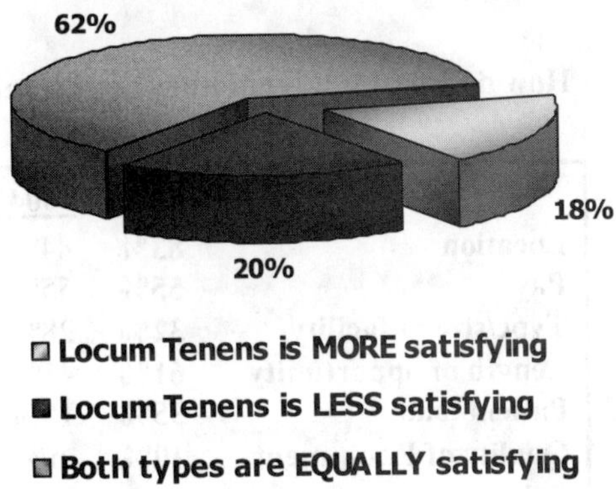

Why Practice Locums?

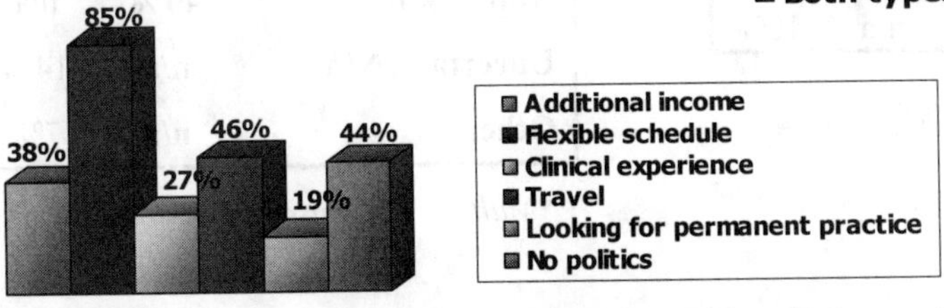

**Asked to indicate all that apply*

What Are The Drawbacks

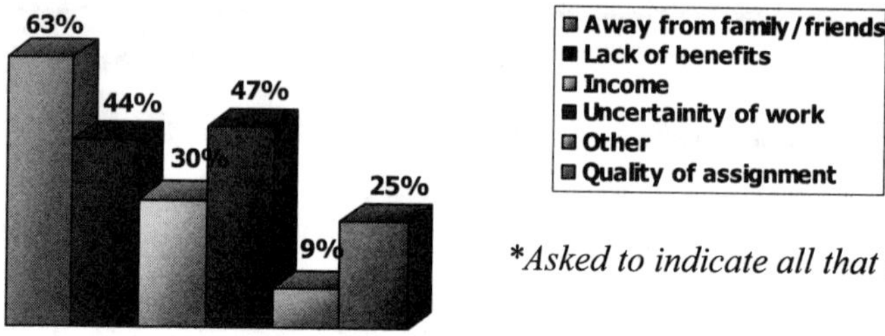

Asked to indicate all that apply

How many staffing firms do you work with?

	2005	2004	2003
None	**6%**	9%	5%
1	**31%**	40%	35%
2-3	**50%**	44%	54%
4 or more	**13%**	7%	6%

Asked to indicate all that apply

How do you choose a firm?

	2005	2004	2003
Pay rate	47%	49%	61%
Reputation/name recognition	42%	28%	31%
Malpractice insurance	32%	21%	24%
Number of opportunities	39%	28%	49%
Location of opportunities	60%	63%	71%
Customer service	57%	45%	n/a
Advertising/Marketing	n/a	4%	5%
Other	11%	15%	3%

How do you select temporary opportunities?

	2005	2004
Location	**83%**	84%
Pay	**55%**	55%
Type/size of facility	**32%**	28%
Length of opportunity	**61%**	45%
Patient load	**35%**	15%
Quality of Equipment	**10%**	n/a
Other	**n/a**	10%

Asked to indicate all that apply

What is your greatest value to the hiring facility?

	2005	2004
To generate revenue	**52%**	15%
To maintain patient care	**87%**	56%
Prevent staff burnout	**56%**	8%
Add a skill	**40%**	n/a
Uncertain, N/A	**n/a**	14%
Other	**n/a**	7%

Multiple responses possible in 2005

What is YOUR perception?

As a locum tenens provider, how do you feel you are viewed by:

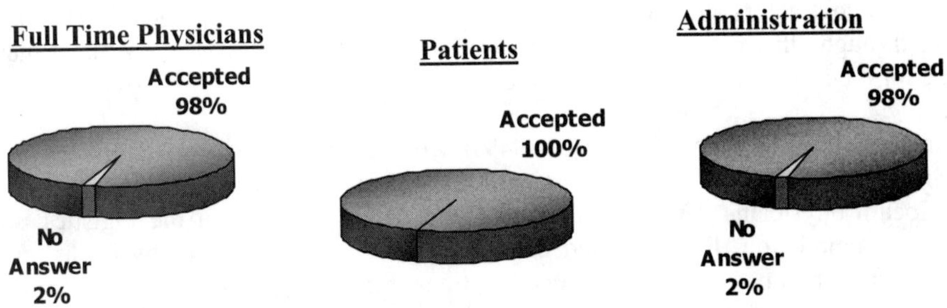

Trends and Observations

Part II of the Review reflects several characteristics of locum tenens physicians surveyed and suggests some of the reasons why they work on a temporary basis.

The majority of locum tenens physicians surveyed (54%) have 21 years or more experience as physicians, up from 43% in 2004's survey grouping. In addition, 36% of those surveyed have three or more years experience working locum tenens, up from 28% in the 2004 survey and 20% in the 2003 survey. While physicians of all experience levels work as locum tenens, the survey sample indicates that physicians working on a temporary basis often have multiple years of medical experience.

The majority of physicians surveyed (57%) work one to three locum tenens assignments per year. About one quarter work 4-6 assignments, while 20% work 7 or more assignments. The ideal assignment length for a large number of those surveyed (50%) is one to 4 months.

The survey indicates that a growing number of physicians view locum tenens as a long-term career option. Over half (51%) indicated they plan to practice on a temporary basis for more than three years, up from 43% last year and 39% the year before. About 18% plan to practice on a temporary basis until they find a permanent position. Among younger physicians, it seems common to use locum tenens to "test drive" various practice settings until they find one that suits their needs.

The majority of those surveyed (63%) are not in a permanent practice, while 37% are working in a permanent position while also working on temporary assignments. Ninety-one percent have worked in a permanent position, while 9% have worked only locum tenens. Of those who have worked in a permanent position, 62% indicate that permanent medical work and temporary work are equally satisfying, while 18% rate locum tenens work as more satisfying than permanent and 20% rate permanent more satisfying than temporary.

When asked why they practice locum tenens, 85% of those surveyed identified "flexible schedule" as a reason, followed by 46% who cited "travel" and 44% who cited "no politics." By contrast, only 38% cited "additional income" as a reason for working locum tenens. For most physicians, locum tenens represents a lifestyle choice and not necessarily a chance to other so-called "hassle-factors" of traditional medicine.

Being away from family and friends is the drawback to locum tenens practice most frequently cited by those surveyed, followed by lack of benefits. Locum tenens physicians are independent contractors and are not employed by temporary staffing agencies. They may get benefits through other permanent employers apart from their locum assignments or they may arrange for their own health insurance and other "benefits."

The great majority of those surveyed (94%) work with at least one temporary staffing company, while 63% work with at least two. Temporary physician staffing companies help match locum physicians with opportunities and arrange for many of the logistics, such as travel, accommodation, licensure and credentialing. Sixty percent of physicians surveyed select staffing firms based on the practice locations they offer, while 57% select firms based on the customer service they provide.

When asked how they select a temporary opportunity, 83% of physicians surveyed identified "location" as a factor, followed by 63% who identified "length of opportunity," and 55% who identified "pay." As independent contractors, locum tenens physicians are able to select which locations they prefer as well as what level of pay they will to accept. If a particular staffing firm is not able to match them with a location they like, they may choose to work through another firm or contract directly with a hospital or medical group.

When asked what value they bring to a medical facility, 87% of locum tenens physicians surveyed identified maintaining patient care as a key factor, followed by preventing staff burnout. Over 50% indicated that they help facilities to generate revenue while 40% indicated they add a clinical skill.

In the early stages of locum tenens practice, dating from the mid-1970's, physicians working locum tenens were not necessarily approved of by their peers, by health care administrators, or by patients. That does not appear to be the case today, however. The great majority of locum tenens physicians interviewed (98%) indicated they are accepted by permanent physicians they work with at their temporary assignments, while 100% said they are accepted by patients, and 98% said they were accepted by administrators.

As the use of locum tenens physicians has become more common, and as privileging requirements and practices have become more stringent, concerns about the quality of care provided by locum tenens physicians seem to have faded.

Review of Staff Care's 2005 Temporary Physician Staffing Assignments

In the course of a calendar year, Staff Care conducts thousands of temporary physician search assignments for its clients, seeking to match independent contractor physicians in multiple specialties with hospitals, medical groups, government facilities and other organizations requiring the services of *locum tenens* physicians.

Following is a review of the temporary physician staffing assignments Staff Care conducted in calendar year 2005. The Review reflects current trends in the locum tenens industry, such as which medical specialties are in the greatest demand and where the demand for temporary physician services appears to be greatest.

Top Temporary Physician Staffing Assignments By Specialty

Days Requested	2005	2004
Family Practice	24%	10%
Anesthesiology/CRNA	24%	32%
Psychiatry	21%	29%
Internal Medicine	12%	7%
Radiology	12%	15%
Pediatrics	2%	3%
Orthopedic Surgery	2%	3%
OBGYN	2%	n/a
General Surgery	n/a	2%

Total Number of Temporary Providers Matched by Staff Care

2006*	2005	2004	2003
8,500	7,600	6,317	5,673

**estimate*

Average Length of Assignment (in days)

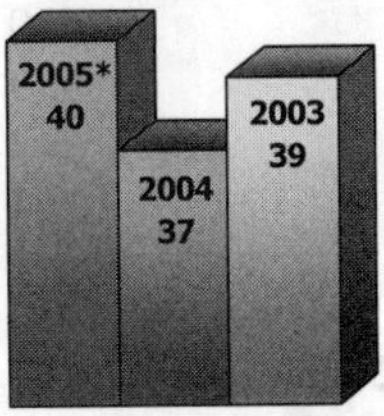

Estimate of Physicians Working Locums Nationally*

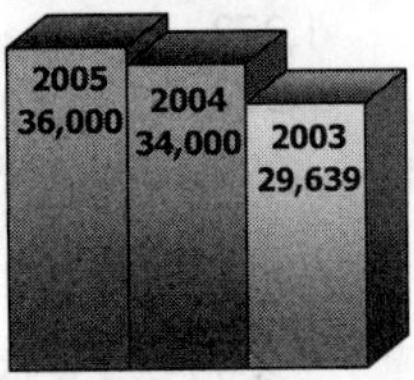

National Spending Estimate (billions) On Temporary Physician Staffing*

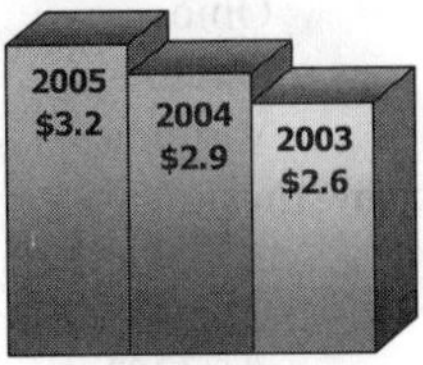

**Based on internal Staff Care data*

Demand for Temporary Physician Staffing Services by State for Specific Specialties

(Based on Physician Days Requested 2005)

Psychiatry

2005		2004	
California	5,487	California	10,745
New York	3,144	Texas	3,921
Texas	3,004	New York	3,019
North Carolina	2,556	Georgia	2,874
Indiana	2,422	Ohio	2,677

Radiology

2005		2004	
New York	3,192	New York	2,082
California	2,988	Florida	1,729
Texas	2,773	Texas	1,394
Pennsylvania	2,618	Georgia	1,301
Florida	2,468	Tennessee	1,156

Orthopedic Surgery

2005		2004	
Minnesota	527	Mississippi	880
South Carolina	425	Minnesota	526
Virginia	375	Washington	517
Indiana	346	Wisconsin	312
Washington	306	Virginia	261

Internal Medicine

2005		2004	
Texas	1,555	Georgia	1,332
Wisconsin	1,235	California	893
California	820	Minnesota	854
Virginia	518	Pennsylvania	836
New Mexico	414	North Carolina	667

Family Practice

2005		2004	
Texas	4,073	California	2,059
California	2,039	Oklahoma	1,630
Ohio	1,272	Georgia	909
Oklahoma	1,232	North Carolina	847
Virginia	805	Missouri	789

Anesthesia | **CRNA**

Anesthesia 2005		CRNA 2005	
Arizona	2,877	North Carolina	6,097
Indiana	1,514	Florida	3,691
Maryland	1,218	Virginia	3,047
New York	837	Texas	2,747
Pennsylvania	778	Pennsylvania	2,728

Anesthesia / CRNA

2004	
Texas	1,555
Wisconsin	1,235
California	820
Virginia	518
New Mexico	414

Trends and Observations

The review of Staff Care's 2005 temporary physician assignments signals several trends of note to health care administrators, health care providers, and others tracking developments in physician staffing.

The Review indicates a dramatic shift in the type of physicians in most demand as locum tenens. In 2004, anesthesiologists and certified registered nurse anesthetists (CRNAs) topped the list of temporary providers in greatest demand among Staff Care's clients, followed by psychiatrists and radiologists. In 2005, the demand for temporary primary care physicians such as family practitioners and general internists increased dramatically, tripling in both specialties, and putting family practice at the top of the "most wanted" list.

Staff Care attributes the rise in demand for primary care as in part a response to the diminishing supply of primary care physicians coming out of residency training. As new physicians gravitate toward more lucrative and less time-intensive specialties, the number of candidates for permanent primary care positions seems to be diminishing, driving the need for temporary physicians to hold a place until a permanent candidate can be found. In addition, for several years hospitals and medical groups have focused on recruiting revenue-generating specialists and now may be playing "catch up" to ensure they have an adequate number of primary care doctors to see patients and make referrals.

Demand for temporary primary care physicians has not diminished demand for other types of doctors, however. The number of days Staff Care clients requested for anesthesiology/CRNA, psychiatry, and radiology all increased in 2005, underlining the generally high demand for physicians across all specialties.

Demand for locum tenens psychiatrists is enhanced by the fact that an increasing volume of psychiatry services are being delivered at correctional facilities. These facilities traditionally have a hard time attracting permanent physicians and often may rely on temporary physicians to maintain services.

While demand for locum tenens services is rising, so is the number of physicians who work on a locum tenens basis. The number of locum tenens providers (physicians and CRNAs) Staff Care matched with temporary assignments grew from 6,317 in 2004 to 7,600 in 2005, an increase of 17%. In 2006, Staff Care matched an estimated 8,500 providers with temporary assignments, an increase of 11% over 2005.

Based in part on the growing number of providers Staff Care is assisting to find temporary assignments, and an understanding of the approximate number of providers other temporary staffing agencies are working with, we estimate some 36,000 physicians practiced on a temporary basis in 2005. This includes an estimate of the number of providers who are arranging for their own temporary assignments directly with hospitals and other health care organizations.

Staff Care further estimates that total annual spending on temporary physician and CRNA services nationwide now exceeds the $3 billion mark. This estimate is based on an understanding of Staff Care's market share in the temporary staffing industry and on an approximation of the number of "physician days" being filled both by agencies and by physicians making direct arrangements with hospitals, medical groups, and other health care organizations. Included in this estimate is spending on "contract management" physician services, such as emergency medicine management or anesthesiology management.

Since 2001, spending on temporary physician services has more than doubled, based on internal estimates, an indication of the growing demand for temporary physician services and the growing number of physicians practicing on a temporary basis.

Other Surveys Available:

- Merritt, Hawkins & Associates® Review of Physician Recruiting Incentives
- Staff Care® Review of Temporary Physician Staffing Trends
- Med Travelers® Review of Temporary Healthcare Staffing Trends and Incentives
- Merritt, Hawkins & Associates® Survey of Final-Year Medical Residents
- Merritt, Hawkins & Associates® Survey of Physicians 50-65 Years Old
- Merritt, Hawkins & Associates® Survey of Inpatient/Outpatient Physician Revenue
- Merritt, Hawkins & Associates® Survey of Physician Appointment Wait Times
- Merritt, Hawkins & Associates® Survey of Primary Care Physicians

ABOUT MERRITT, HAWKINS & ASSOCIATES AND AMN HEALTHCARE

Established in 1987, Merritt, Hawkins & Associates is the nation's leading physician search and consulting firm. Merritt, Hawkins & Associates was formerly part of The MHA Group of healthcare staffing companies, which also included:

Staff Care. Staff Care is the leading temporary (i.e., *locum tenens)* physician staffing firm in the United States.

Med Travelers. Med Travelers is one of the largest allied health professional staffing firms in the United States.

RN Demand. RN Demand is a leading temporary nurse staffing firm.

In 2005, The MHA Group merged with AMN Healthcare, Inc., to create the nation's largest health care staffing firm. With over 2,000 employees and offices located throughout the United States and internationally, AMN Healthcare, Inc. provides services in nurse, physician and allied health care professional staffing.

For additional information, please contact:

Merritt, Hawkins & Associates
A Division of AMN Healthcare, Inc.
5001 Statesman Drive
Irving, Texas 75063
800-876-0500
469-524-1400
www.mhagroup.com

Notes

Notes

Notes

Notes

Notes